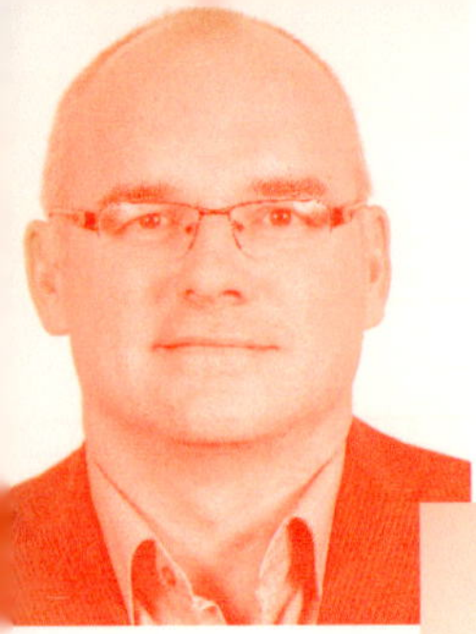
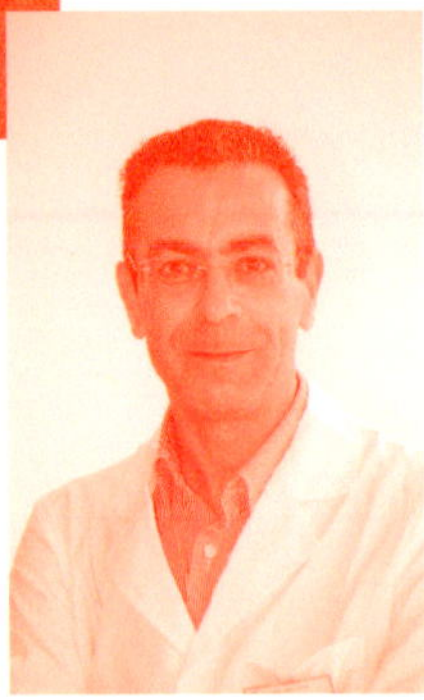
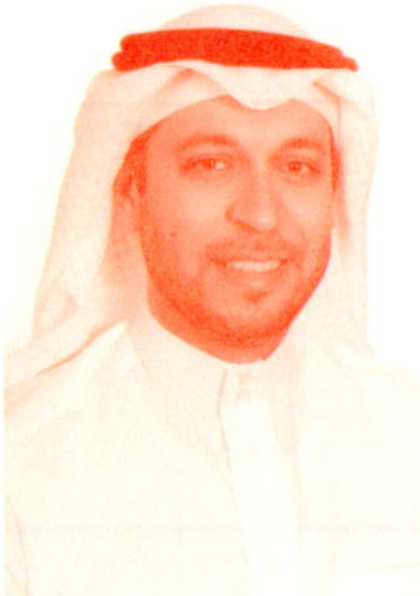
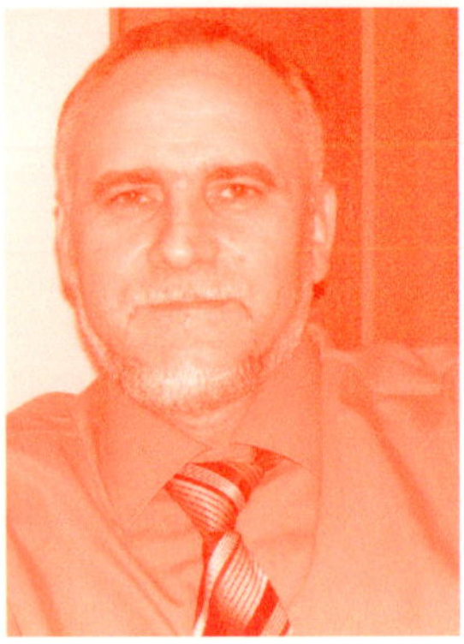
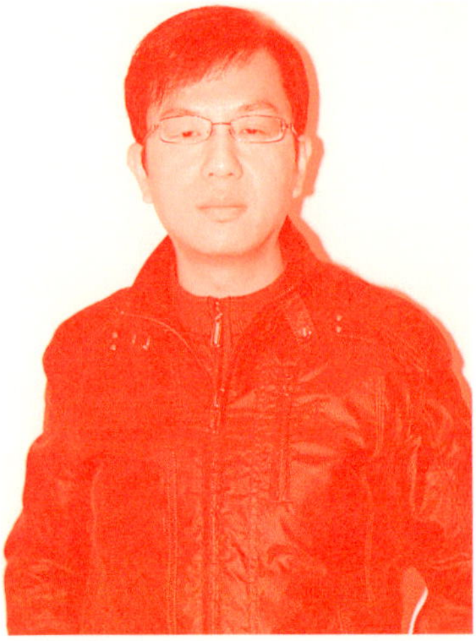
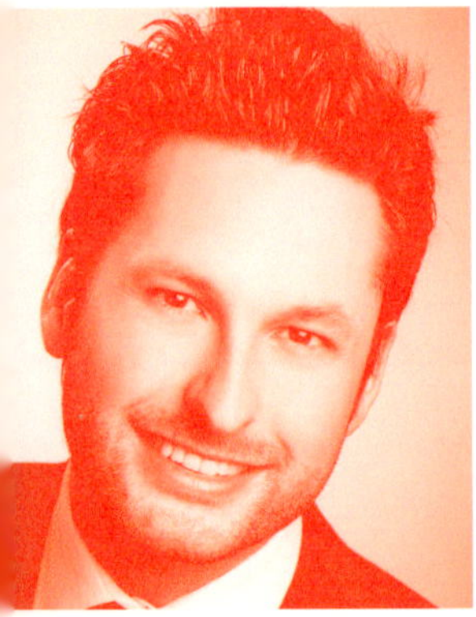
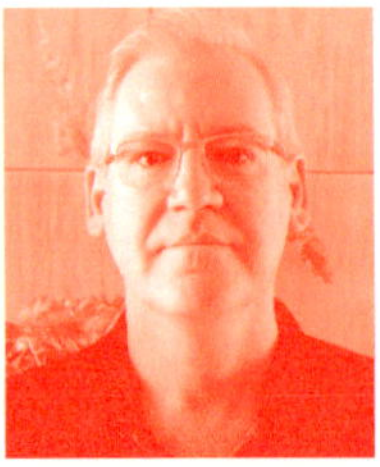

IntechOpen

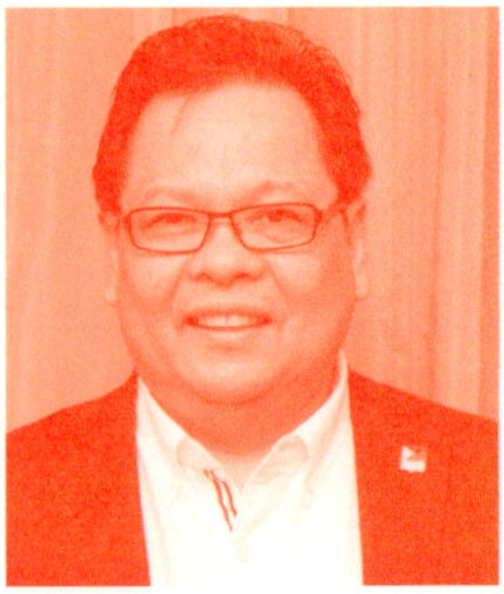
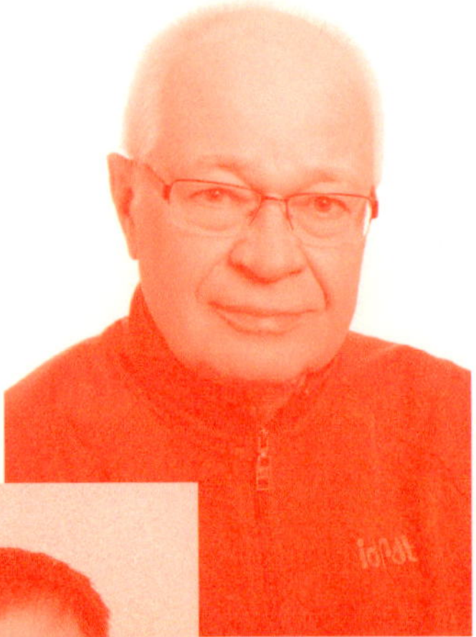
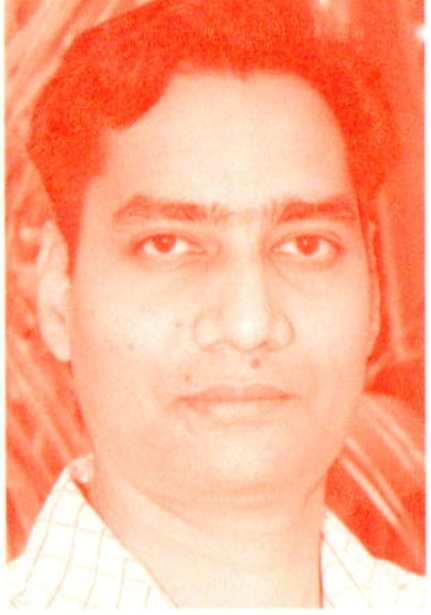
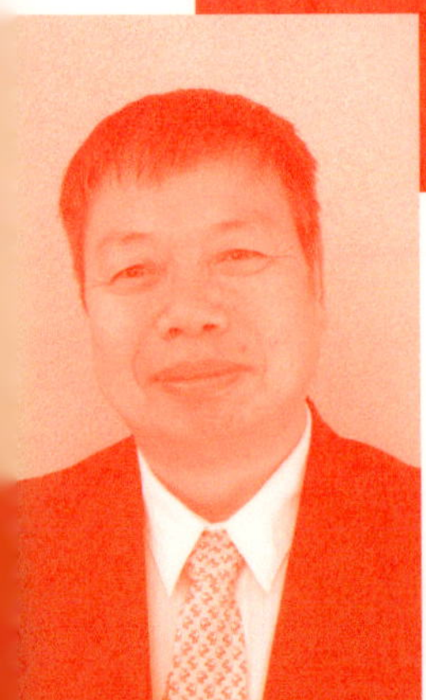
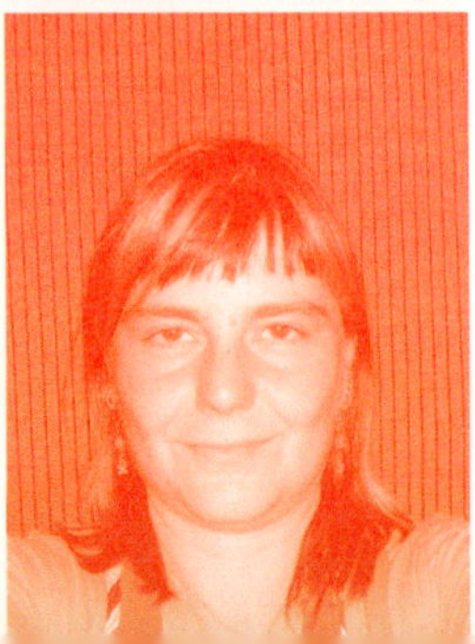
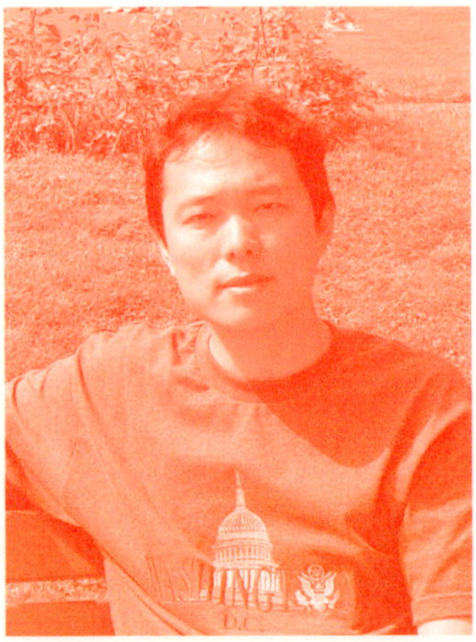

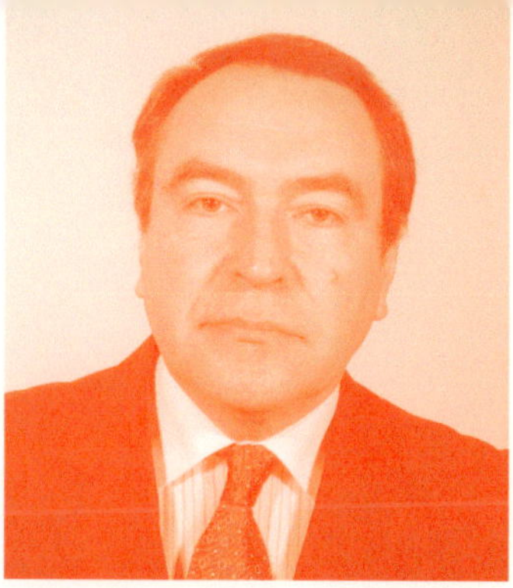
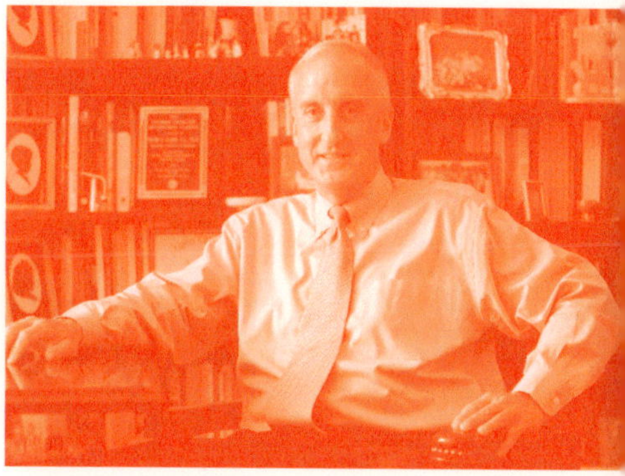
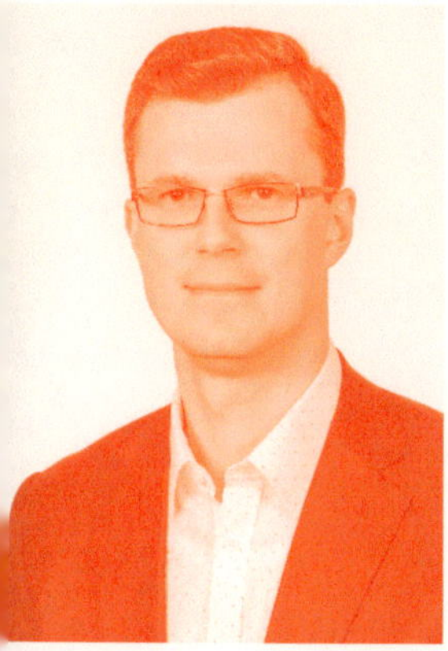
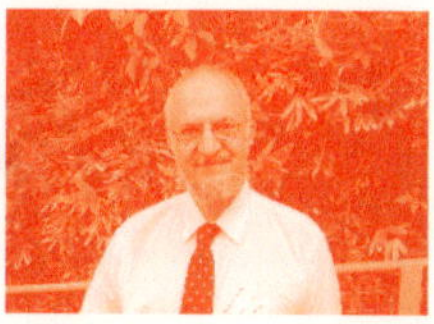
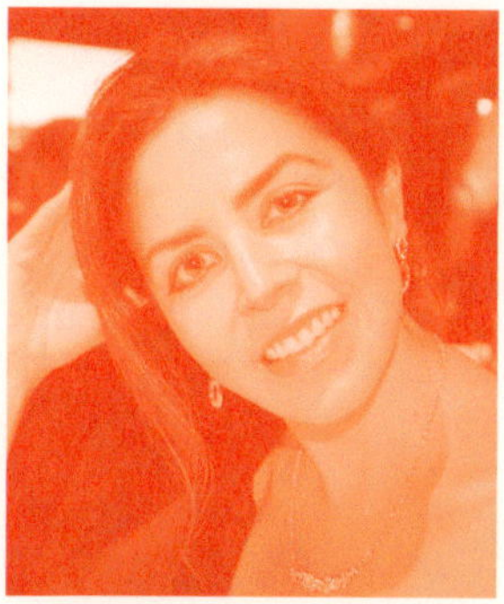

Supporting open minds since 2005

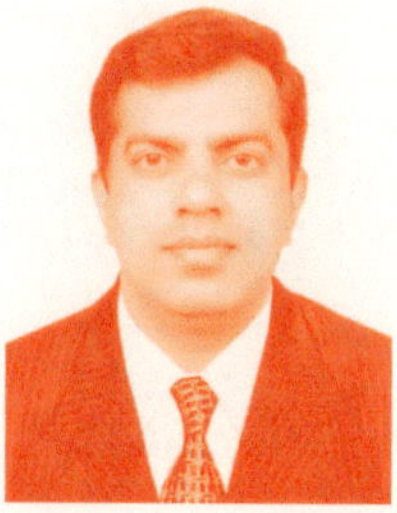
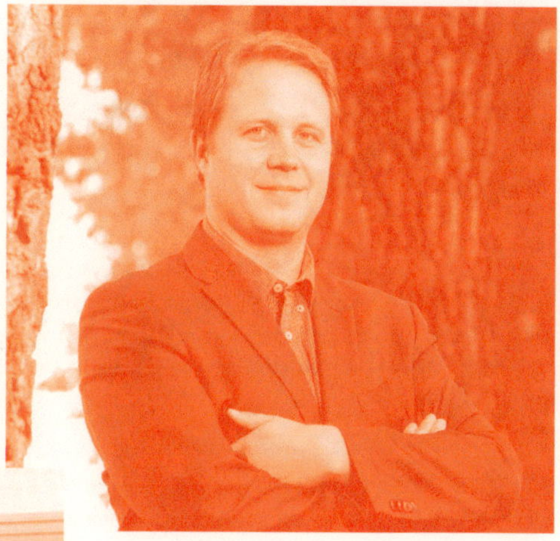
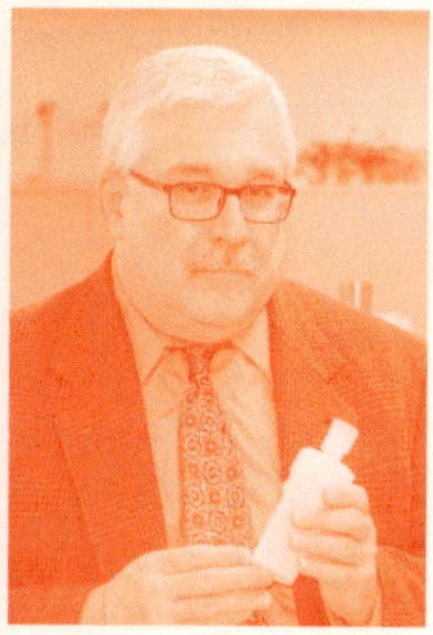
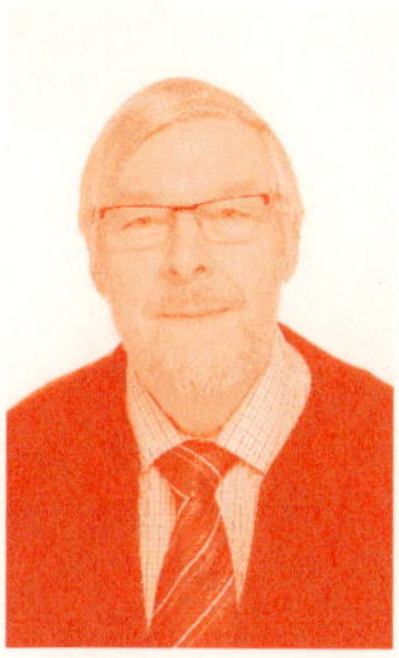
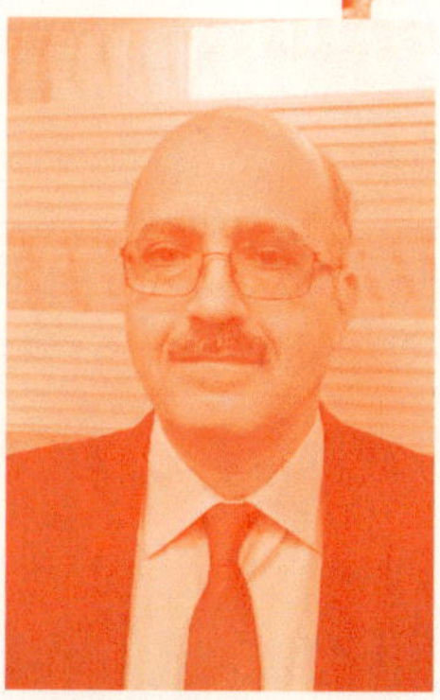
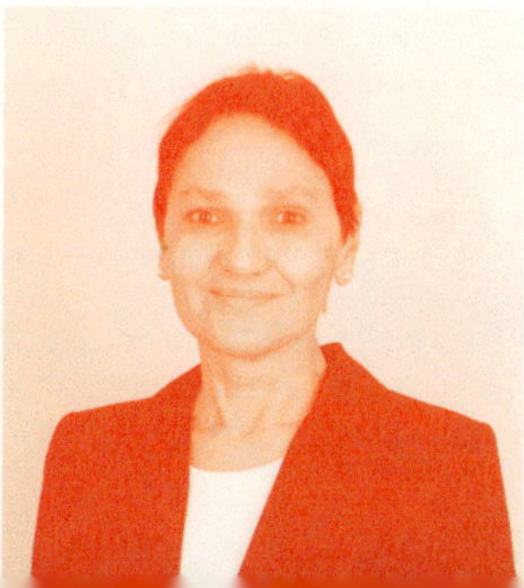
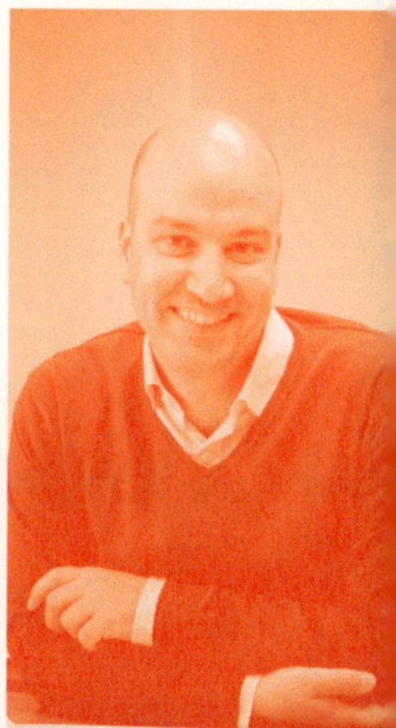

Current Topics in Faecal Incontinence
http://dx.doi.org/10.5772/intechopen.77679
Edited by John Camilleri-Brennan

Contributors
Khalil Bitar, Prabhash Dadhich, Kasaya Tantiphlachiva, Batool Mutar Mahdi, Dimitrios Linardoutsos, Arantxa Muñoz-Duyos, Yolanda Ribas, John Camilleri-Brennan

First published in London, United Kingdom, 2020 by IntechOpen
IntechOpen is the global imprint of INTECHOPEN LIMITED, registered in England and Wales, registration number: 11086078, 7th floor, 10 Lower Thames Street, London, EC3R 6AF, United Kingdom
Printed in Croatia

British Library Cataloguing-in-Publication Data
A catalogue record for this book is available from the British Library

Additional hard and PDF copies can be obtained from orders@intechopen.com

Current Topics in Faecal Incontinence
Edited by John Camilleri-Brennan
p. cm.
Print ISBN 978-1-78984-325-5
Online ISBN 978-1-78984-326-2
eBook (PDF) ISBN 978-1-83880-328-5

For EU product safety concerns:
IN TECH d.o.o., Prolaz Marije Krucifikse Kozulić 3, 51000 Rijeka, Croatia, info@intechopen.com or visit our website at intechopen.com.

Meet the editor

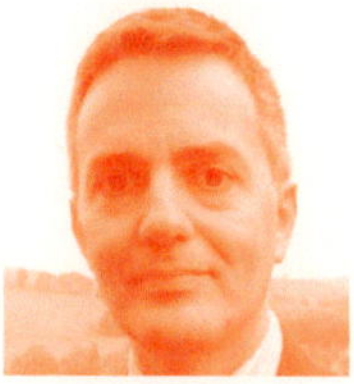

John Camilleri-Brennan MD (Melit), MD (Dundee), FRCSGlas, FRCSGenSurg, MFSTEd is a consultant in general and colorectal surgery and colorectal clinical lead with NHS Forth Valley in Scotland, and honorary clinical associate professor with the University of Glasgow. A graduate of the University of Malta, he received his postgraduate surgical training primarily in Dundee and Aberdeen. A travelling fellowship by the Royal College of Physicians and Surgeons of Glasgow enabled him to pursue further studies in colorectal surgery at the University of Minnesota, USA. His research on rectal cancer led to a doctorate from the University of Dundee. He is the recipient of the William Cullen Prize from the Royal College of Physicians of Edinburgh for his work on faecal incontinence.

Contents

Preface

Faecal incontinence is, for the majority, a physically debilitating and socially stigmatising condition that may have quite a profound adverse effect on one's quality of life, it being associated with poor self-esteem, embarrassment, and depression. The causes are multifactorial, the investigations are varied, and the treatment involves a multidisciplinary team of professionals who work with patients and their significant others to optimise the quality of their lives. The treatment modalities range from simple measures and lifestyle modifications to complex interventions.

This book, *Current Topics in Faecal Incontinence*, features an international authorship. The clinicians and researchers who contributed to this book have a wealth of experience and have made seminal contributions to their respective fields. The chapters represent both original research as well as up-to-date and comprehensive reviews. The clinical, anatomical, and physiological evaluation of faecal incontinence, including quality of life, is discussed in some detail. Chapters are also devoted to faecal incontinence in autoimmune disease and obstructive defaecation. The final two chapters focus on two key and expanding areas in the treatment of faecal incontinence: anal implants and biosphincters.

This book should appeal to a wide readership. It is an invaluable resource for physicians, surgeons, nurses, and allied healthcare professionals who seek to refresh and expand their knowledge in this field, as well as a source of excellent information for those preparing for professional examinations. I trust that readers will find this book both enjoyable as well as educationally rewarding.

I hope that, with this book, I have contributed in some way to the understanding of this complex yet common condition, and ultimately provide a service that will benefit patients and improve their quality of life. I am most grateful to the authors who have willingly put in an enormous effort in providing such excellent reviews of these diverse topics.

John Camilleri-Brennan MD (Melit), MD (Dundee), FRCSGlas, FRCSGenSurg, MFSTEd
University of Glasgow,
Glasgow, Scotland, UK

Section 1

Introduction

Chapter 1

Introductory Chapter: Challenges in the Diagnosis and Treatment of Faecal Incontinence

John Camilleri-Brennan

1. Introduction

Faecal incontinence is defined as the involuntary loss of faeces and flatus through the anal canal and the inability to postpone defaecation until socially convenient. In the majority, it is a physically debilitating and socially stigmatising condition that may have an adverse effect on one's quality of life. There are many aspects of one's life that are affected by this condition. Faecal incontinence has been shown to be associated with poor self-esteem, embarrassment, and depression. Those afflicted with this condition frequently need to plan and organise their lives around the availability of and easy access to bathrooms and frequently avoid social and leisure activities, especially venturing outdoors.

The prevalence of faecal incontinence in the UK is estimated to be about 2% of the general population. Certainly the prevalence increases with age. Other independent risk factors include female sex, physical limitations, poor general health, and loose and frequent stools. From the financial point of view, the investigation and treatment of faecal incontinence may add to a significant cost to the health budget of most countries. In fact, the annual cost to treat and care for patients in the UK with urinary and faecal incontinence and the consequences thereof is of about £500 million. In addition, there are significant financial costs to the patients, their families, and their employers due to the time taken off work and unemployment.

1.1 Diagnostic challenges

The pathophysiology of faecal incontinence is multifactorial. This presents the first challenge: that of reaching a correct diagnosis. A thorough clinical assessment of the patient is therefore mandatory. A detailed history, including a cognitive assessment in most cases, is necessary. The characteristics of the faeces and the type and frequency of incontinence should be noted. Urge incontinence is suggestive of poor external anal sphincter function, whilst passive and post-defaecatory incontinence indicates that internal anal sphincter function is weak. Any red flag symptoms, the symptoms suggestive of colorectal cancer such as rectal bleeding, should be identified. Importance should be placed on secondary symptoms such as pruritus ani and perianal skin, since these may reflect upon the severity of the incontinence and may in some cases be the presenting complaint. Various questionnaires that enable the clinician to quantify the degree of incontinence, the severity of symptoms, and the impact on quality of life are available. These include symptom-specific questionnaires, such as the ones developed by Vaizey et al. [1] and Jorge and Wexner [2], the Fecal Incontinence Quality of Life Scale (FIQOL) developed

IntechOpen

by Rockwood et al. [3], and also generic questionnaires such as the Short Form 36 (SF 36) [4]. Further information is obtained from a full examination of the patient, including the abdomen and perineum, and a neurological examination in some cases. Beneficial investigations include a flexible sigmoidoscopy, anal manometry (resting and squeeze pressure), rectal compliance, pudendal nerve terminal motor latency (PNTML), endoanal ultrasound, and defaecating proctography. Clinicians, however, need to be able to determine which test to perform and when. Crucially important is the correct interpretation of the results to ensure as accurate a diagnosis as possible. This presents a difficulty in itself due to our incomplete knowledge in some areas of physiology and pathophysiology and also due to the weak correlation between subjective and objective parameters.

1.2 Treatment challenges

The treatment of faecal incontinence is most often demanding. Determining the appropriate treatment depends upon the accuracy of the diagnosis but also has to be tailored to the individual patient, taking into consideration the individual circumstances.

There are many publications listing the various modalities of conservative and operative treatment options. The main aim is to treat the patients' incontinence conservatively in the first instance. Stool consistency may be improved with the use of loperamide and codeine, biofeedback and pelvic floor exercises may help improve rectal evacuation, anal plugs minimise passive incontinence, and so on. Failure of medical therapy may lead to consideration of surgical options, of which a variety are available. For example, traumatic disruption to the anal sphincter and pelvic floor may be repaired, either by simple muscle apposition or, in exceptional circumstances, by more advanced and complex techniques such as the gracilis neosphincter. However, direct surgery on the colon, rectum, and anal sphincter is both invasive and irreversible, as well as being associated with poorly sustained long-term outcomes and well-established complications. A less invasive surgical mode of treatment is sacral nerve stimulation (SNS), which has been shown to be effective in the improvement of continence in a selected group of patients. Other more minimally invasive procedures, such as the SECCA procedure and the use of anal bulking agents, have an important role to play. Scientific advances in the field of anal implants, with their associated clinical benefits and safety profile, are making these minimally invasive operations a more viable and effective option. A colostomy always remains an option and may be considered in certain circumstances, such as in those who are bed-bound, those with upper motor neurone lesions, and those where other surgical options have failed or are considered inappropriate.

The choice of treatment is not always straightforward. It is therefore advisable that patients are managed in a multidisciplinary setting, especially those who failed conservative management and may require operative intervention. Continence multidisciplinary team meetings to discuss patients with challenging continence issues are therefore highly commended [5].

Moving forwards, we are faced with exciting challenges as technology is rapidly advancing. A main example is the intrinsically innervated BioSphincter, which has the potential to improve the quality of life of so many of our patients. Watch this space!

Author details

John Camilleri-Brennan
University of Glasgow, UK

*Address all correspondence to: johncbrennan@doctors.org.uk

References

[1] Vaizey CJ, Carapeti E, Cahill JA, Kamm MA. Prospective comparison of faecal incontinence grading systems. Gut. 1999;**44**:77-80

[2] Jorge JMN, Wexner SD. Etiology and management of faecal incontinence. Diseases of the Colon and Rectum. 1993;**36**:77-97

[3] Rockwood TH, Church JM, Fleshman JW, et al. Fecal incontinence quality of life scale: Quality of life instrument for patients with fecal incontinence. Diseases of the Colon and Rectum. 2000;**43**(1):9-17

[4] Ware JE Jr, Sherbourne CD. The MOS 36-item short-form health survey (SF-36). I. Conceptual framework and item selection. Medical Care. 1992;**30**:473-483

[5] National Institute for Clinical Excellence (NICE). The Management of Faecal Incontinence in Adults. Clinical Guideline 49 NICE 2007

Section 2

Clinical Anatomical and Physiological Evaluation

Chapter 2

Comprehensive Clinical Approach to Fecal Incontinence

Kasaya Tantiphlachiva

Abstract

Fecal incontinence is a disturbing condition, which reduces the quality of life of patients. Prevalence of this apprehensive problem is usually underestimated. However, it is more common in female, elderly, and institutionalized subjects. Factors that may be associated are urinary incontinence, diabetes mellitus, depression, diarrhea, history of anorectal surgery, anorectal trauma, pelvic organ surgery, and pelvic irradiation. To improve this condition, physicians should have insight into the individual's pathophysiology through the process of careful history taking, severity, and quality of life assessment, thorough physical examination and comprehensive anatomic and neurophysiologic evaluation. These tests include imaging, anorectal manometry, and neural conduction tests. Finally, by these gathered information, individualized treatment for the patient is designed. Patient's education and judicious follow-up are also parts of the plan.

Keywords: fecal incontinence, digital rectal examination, endoanal ultrasound, anorectal manometry, neurophysiologic test

1. Introduction

Fecal incontinence (FI) is defined as recurrent uncontrolled passage of solid or liquid stool at least 3 months in an at least 4-year-old individual [1]. For research, onset should be at least 6 months with the episodes of two times in 4 week-period [1]. Severity of FI has a direct deteriorating effect on the quality of life of the patients, especially on life style and depression [2, 3]. The higher severity was also significantly associated with more direct annual medical (i.e. medical resources used for diagnosis, treatment, and management of related conditions) and nonmedical costs (i.e. nonmedical care such as transportation and use of protective products) [4]. Other indirect cost is associated with loss of productivity [4] and work load of caregivers [5]. Prevalence of FI in general population was 7.7% (range, 2.0–20.7%) [6, 7]. It equally affected both gender in most studies; male 8.1% (range 2.3–16.1%) and female 8.9% (range 2.0–20.7%) [7, 8]. The prevalence increased with age, that is, 5.7% at 15–34 year, 9.9% at 60–90 year, and 15.9% at >90 years [7, 9]. Associated risk factors of FI included increasing age, watery stool, functional diarrhea, urinary incontinence, and polypharmacy (use of five or more medications) [5, 7, 9, 10, 11]. In instituted population, the prevalence of FI was up to 46–57.1% [11, 12]. Significant associated factors of FI were poor general health status (≥4 comorbidities), urinary incontinence, cognitive-function impairment (dementia), decreased mobility, and length of nursing home residency [12]. In elderly female, marriage was another predictive factor of FI [9]. This may be explained by the difference in pathophysiology of FI in female where parity, traumatic vaginal delivery, and previous pelvic surgery played roles [13]. In parous female, the incidence of FI was as high as 46% from postal survey [14]. In male with FI, impaired rectal sensation and evacuation disorder are more prominent than female [13]. Thus, pathophysiology of FI is likely to be different between genders and individuals. Careful systematic evaluation should be performed to assess these underlying mechanisms in order to guide a successful management.

2. Pathophysiology of fecal incontinence

Normal control of defecation requires intact neuromuscular structures, including rectum, anal canal, pelvic floor, and neural network. Rectum, as a reservoir; anal canal, with intact sensation and vascular cushion as a checkpoint; pelvic floor and anal sphincter, as controlling gate; and neural network, as a communication system, all play roles in bowel control. For perfect action, colorectal motility, stool volume, and stool consistency should also be normal. Disruption of one or more compositions of the system leads to FI. In clinical practice, most patients with FI were found to have multiple contributing factors [15].

Rectum is the distal part of colon, which extends from the rectosigmoid junction, dilates to form a reservoir, and ends at the tight circular anal canal [16]. It is distensible and acts as a temporary storage of residue of ingested food [17]. Surgical removal of rectum or physical injury to rectum such as radiation predisposes the subject to FI.

Anal canal is the terminal part of the gastrointestinal tract. It is a close tube surrounded by anal sphincter muscle (surgical anal canal). Anal sphincter and pelvic floor muscle act together to close the bowel. Anal sphincter muscles comprise internal anal sphincter (IAS) and external anal sphincter (EAS). ***IAS*** is the inner circular smooth muscle layer, which contributes to most of the anal sphincter pressure at rest [17, 18]. It is a continuation of inner circular muscle of the rectum and ends just proximal to the subcutaneous part of EAS [18]. Its length is 2.5 cm and thickness is 2–5 mm in normal population [18]. IAS is innervated by the autonomic nervous system. Parasympathetic supply is from the first, second, and third sacral nerves via pelvic plexus and sympathetic supply from both thoracolumbar outflow and hypogastric nerves [18]. The enteric nervous system connecting between neurons and glial cells situates in the myenteric (Auerbach's) plexus and the submucosal (Meissner's) plexus is a part of reflex pathways that control bowel [18]. ***EAS*** is the outer striated muscle layer, which voluntarily functions during squeeze. In the literature, it had been described as three parts: subcutaneous, superficial, and deep [19, 20]. However, the findings during surgery and from advance imaging, the current concept accepts that the deep portion of EAS it on continuous circumferential mass with the puborectalis muscle [19]. The upper part of superficial EAS is attached anteriorly with transverse perinei muscle at the perineal body [19]. The subcutaneous portion of EAS is just underneath the skin and is traversed by the conjoined longitudinal muscle, which is the continuation of the outer longitudinal layer of the rectum. EAS is innervated by the perineal branch of pudendal nerve (S2–4), inferior rectal nerve, and perineal branch of the forth sacral nerve [19, 21]. These nerves contribute in various patterns [21]. Mucosa of the upper anal canal is lined by columnar epithelium and the lower anal canal is lined by squamous epithelium [19]. Submucosal tissue and subepithelial tissue contain internal hemorrhoidal plexus and external hemorrhoidal plexus, respectively [19]. This distensible hemorrhoidal cushion plays a protecting role for anus and helps in complete closure of the anal canal. It contributes to 15–20% of resting anal canal pressure in addition to the major 85% contributed by IAS [22].

Pelvic floor muscle, or the levator ani muscle, continues with the uppermost part of the external anal sphincter. It comprises of (1) *puborectalis muscle*, a U-shaped muscular sling from each side of pubic symphysis that joins behind the rectum at the anorectal junction [17]. It is a major muscle that maintains anorectal angle approximately 90° at rest [19, 22]. (2) *Pubococcygeus muscle*: originates from the back of the pubic bone, lateral to the puborectalis muscles, and from the anterior half of the obturator fascia [19, 22]. It runs backward, downward, and medially to decussate with the fibers from the opposite side forming a tendinous center called anococcygeal raphe [19, 22]. (3) Iliococcygeus muscle arises from the ischial spine and posterior part of the obturator fascia and passes downward, backward, and medially to insert on the lower part of sacrum, coccyx, and anococcygeal raphe [19]. In the middle of the anterior part of the levator ani, there is the levator hiatus, which pelvic organs pass through [19]. Pubococcygeus and iliococcygeus contribute to lateral pressure to narrow the levator hiatus, and puborectalis muscle has a role in maintaining continence [22]. Impaired levator ani contraction is strongly correlated with severity of FI [23]. Levator ani is innervated by direct branches from sacral nerves (S3–5) proximal to sacral plexus [19, 24].

Sensory innervation of the anorectal area is responsible for correct afferent information of the luminal content. Anal canal is sensitive to pain, temperature, and touch, and afferent conduction is via pudendal nerve back to S2, S3, and S4 nerve roots [16, 25]. For rectum, parasympathetic fiber transmits the sensation of rectal distension via the nervi erigentes which are derived from the S2, S3, and S4 spinal segment [22]. These fibers join the sympathetic nerve fiber which is derived from L1, L2, and L3 spinal segment [16, 18, 22, 24] to form hypogastric plexus [18, 24].

Sacral reflexes, including rectoanal inhibitory reflex (RAIR), sampling reflex, and cough reflex, are additional mechanisms of sensing and controlling stool [26]. These involve anorectum sensing area, peripheral nerve, spinal cord sensory and motor nuclei, and anorectal musculature, acting in a coordinated circle. ***RAIR***, mediated by intramural myenteric neurons, is an immediate IAS relaxation following rectal distension [26]. Sensation of rectal distention and stretch by nerve fibers in rectal mucosa, submucosa, and myenteric plexus then go along the parasympathetic system to S2, S3, and S4 [27]. When the intrarectal pressure becomes higher than intra-anal canal pressure, bowel content is allowed to reach the anodermal area in the upper anal canal where sensory receptors are abundant [26, 27]. This anorectal sampling reflex provides information for discrimination between solid, liquid, and gas contents [27]. Thus, the person can choose to retain those contents in the bowel or pass it out at an appropriate time.

Cough reflex prevents leakage during a sudden rise in intra-abdominal pressure by immediate contraction of EAS [26]. It is triggered by receptors on the pelvic floor and transferred through a spinal reflex arc [28]. Connection between the central nervous system and the anorectal area contributes to a higher function of bowel control. Intact CNS to percept, process, and produce the efferent action is required for perfect control. Specific sensory areas in the brain are responsible for sensing the rectal distension [29]. Specific motor area in the parasagittal cortex is responsible for controlling anal sphincter [30, 31]. **Figure 1** shows the anatomical and neural pathways of fecal continence control.

FI occurs when one or more of the controlling mechanisms were damaged. Obvious etiology of FI is anal sphincter damage. In females, obstetric anal sphincter injury can occur after vaginal delivery. Postpartum fecal incontinence had been reported in 3–4% of women [32]. Sphincter weakness after delivery may be caused by injury to internal and external sphincter and injury to pudendal nerve or combination [32]. Risk factors include forcep delivery, prolonged second stage of labor (>5 h), shoulder dystocia, ano-vulvar distance <2 cm, perineal scar and third or

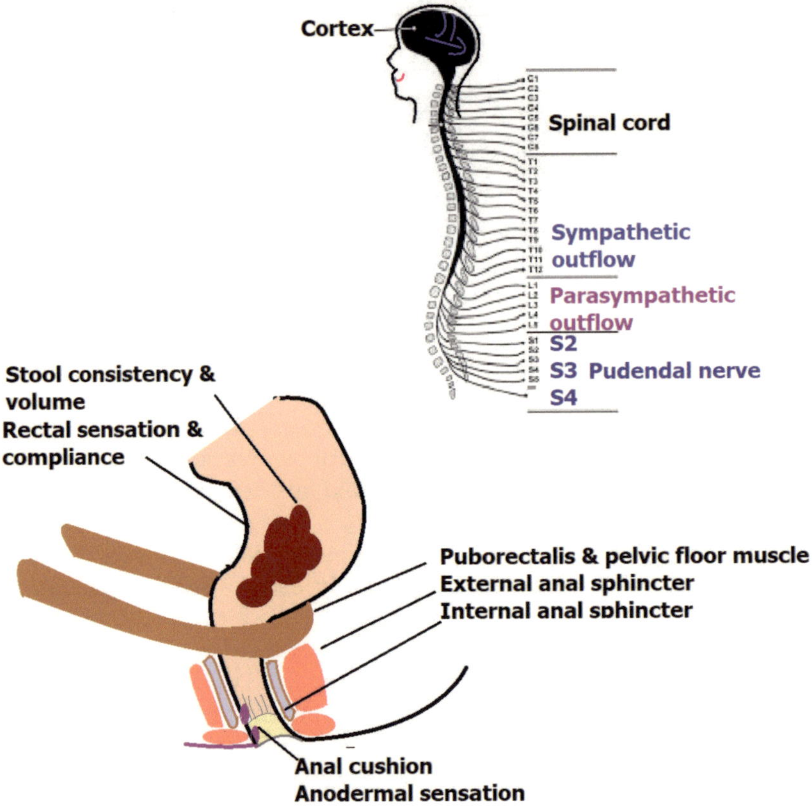

Figure 1.
Fecal continence system.

fourth-degree perineal injury, and infant birth weight >3500 g [32, 33]. Symptoms of continence may occur later in life as there are other compensatory mechanisms to compensate [32]. Symptomatic group was older, had less body mass index, and had more forceps delivery than the asymptomatic group [33]. FI in men was more associated with constipation and previous colon and anorectal surgery compared to women [34]. Anorectal surgery, including hemorrhoidectomy, lateral internal sphincterotomy, and fistulectomy, may affect the anal sphincter and vascular cushion, thus leading to FI [15, 35].

Normal rectum is a low-pressure space acting as a reservoir of fecal material until a coordinated and effective evacuation is appropriate [36]. Decreased rectal compliance, accommodation, or sensation may be found in inflammatory bowel disease and radiation proctitis [15, 36]. Neurological interruption of the central, peripheral, or autonomic nervous system is another cause of FI. These include cerebrovascular accident, spinal cord injury, and pudendal neuropathy. The latter had been reported after radiotherapy for prostatic cancer [37]. FI after multimodality treatment of pelvic malignancy, including prostate, cervical cancer, and rectal cancer, had been reported between 3 and 53% [38].

Other contributing risk factors of FI are stool consistency and transit function of the colon. In the presence of diarrhea and history of previous cholecystectomy, the control of stool becomes more difficult. In obesity, increased body mass index predisposed the subjects to FI due to weakening of pelvic floor musculature and increased intra-abdominal pressure [15, 39]. Shorter anal canal length, lower resting pressure, and higher rectal perception threshold were seen compared to nonobese patients [39]. **Table 1** summarizes the risk factors of fecal incontinence.

Category	Risk factors
Intestinal factors	
	Diarrheal status
	Irritable bowel syndrome
	Inflammatory bowel disease
	Post cholecystectomy
	Malabsorption/food intolerance/enteral tube feeding
	Hypersecretory tumors
Rectal factors	
-Acquired structural abnormalities	Rectal intussusception/rectal prolapse
	Rectal resection
	Trauma/anorectal impalement
	Radiation proctitis
	Ulcerative proctitis
-Overflow	Fecal impaction (overflow incontinence/paradoxical diarrhea)
	Dyssynergic defecation
	Rectal hyposensitivity
Anal sphincter and pelvic floor factors	
-Acquired anatomical defect	Sphincter injury: obstetric, anorectal surgery, accident (e.g. pelvic fracture), and impalement
-Congenital defect	Imperforated anus, cloacal defect, and spina bifida (myelomeningocele and meningocele)
Neurological factors	
-Central nervous system	Cerebrovascular disease
	Trauma brain injury
	Neoplasm of brain and spinal cord
	Cerebral infection
	Multiple sclerosis
	Spinal surgery
	Spina bifida
	Dementia
	Tabes dorsalis
-Peripheral nervous system	Pudendal neuropathy (radiation, diabetes, and chemotherapy)
-Autonomic nervous system	Diabetes mellitus
	Parkinson's disease
	Previous pelvic surgery/radiation
Metabolic and systemic factors	
Endocrine	Diabetic gastroenteropathy and hyperthyroidism
Electrolyte disturbance	Hypercalcemia and hypermagnesemia
Medication	*Causing loose stool:* laxatives/metformin/magnesium-containing antacids/ serotonin reuptake inhibitors, and orlistat
	Alter gut flora: cephalosporins, penicillins, and erythromycin
	Alter sphincter tone: nitrate, calcium channel blocker, sildenafil, and bolulinum toxin injection

Category	Risk factors
Psychological factors	
	Psychiatric disorder
	Medication
Individual characteristics	
	Aging
	Female gender
	Smoking
	Obesity
	Institutionalization/physical disabilities

Table 1.
Risk factors of fecal incontinence.

3. Assessment of fecal incontinence

To define the underlying etiology of FI in each patient, the clinician should have stepwise systematic assessment. There are three important steps in evaluation of patients with FI: clinical assessment, anatomical assessment, and neurophysiologic assessment.

3.1 Clinical assessment

Manifestation of FI may be classified into three subtypes: urge incontinence, total incontinence, and seepage [27].

1. *Passive incontinence*: involuntary leakage of fecal material or gas without awareness.

2. *Urge incontinence:* leakage of fecal material or gas in spite of active attempts to retain them.

3. *Fecal seepage*: undesired leakage of fecal material after normal bowel movement without abnormal continence or evacuation.

Careful history taking should detect patients with FI who may not admit this embarrassing condition [40]. By using different terms, such as diarrhea, fecal urgency, accident, etc., and privacy of the clinic environment should allow more patients to discuss about their symptoms. Information retrieved from history taking should include severity, onset duration, clinical subtypes, and associated symptoms, for example, rectal prolapse, pelvic organ prolapse, and urinary incontinence [41]. Stool diary and stool form charts such as the Bristol stool form scale can be used for better communication [15]. Aggravating factors should be elicited. These include detailed obstetric history and abdominal-colon-anorectal surgical history, and coexisting medical condition should be noted [41]. Previous and current treatments and results should be recorded [41]. Severity score should be documented by using one of the available established scores: St. Mark's Fecal Incontinence Severity Score (Vaizey's score), Cleveland Clinic Fecal Incontinence Score (Wexner's score), the American Medical System score, and Pescatori score [42]. From the international survey, the Wexner score is the most commonly used scoring system even though the score does not include fecal urgency [43]. These scores do not have a cut-off point, may not be used to guide treatment, and cannot predict the treatment outcome [44, 45]. However, it reveals the patient's current

Onset, duration, and precipitating event(s)
Severity and timing of symptoms
Clinical subtypes: passive, urge, and fecal seepage
Clinical grading of severity
Previous and current bowel movement activity; frequency, stool consistency, urgency, change in bowel habit, constipation, and fecal impaction
Coexisting problem: urinary incontinence and pelvic organ prolapses
Previous surgery: anorectal surgery, abdominal surgery, and pelvic surgery
Previous pelvic irradiation
Central nervous system problem: cerebrovascular disease and spinal cord injury
Underlying medical problem and current medication
Current medication/caffeine/diet
Obstetric history: previous delivery, instrumentation, baby birth weight, perineal tear, and repair

Table 2.
Information that should be obtained during history taking from patient with fecal incontinence.

burden which can be used to compare during follow-up after treatment. **Table 2** shows the information that should be obtained during history taking [27]. Change in bowel habit, stool character, advanced age, bleeding per rectum, anemia, mucous bloody stool, and family history of cancer should alert the physician to further endoluminal investigation. Multi-compartment involvement of pelvic organ prolapse should be approached by the multidisciplinary team. Quality of life assessment using standardized scores—fecal incontinence quality of life scale (FIQL) [46], SF-36 (short Medical Outcomes Questionnaire), and Gastrointestinal Quality of Life Index—may be used for clinical assessment and should be used routinely in research [44, 45].

Physical examination, especially perineal and anorectal examination, is an important part of assessment. Information of baseline anatomy and function of the subject are obtained [41]. Patients are usually placed on a left lateral position with hip and knee flexion. ***Inspection*** of the perineum, at rest and strain, may be positive for scar from previous surgery or obstetric injury, skin inflammation, thinning or loss of perineal body, anal gaping, soiling fistula, hemorrhoid, mucosal prolapse, rectal prolapse, and perineal descent [41, 47–49]. Following inspection, ***testing for perineal sensation*** and anocutaneous reflex is performed by stroking the perianal skin in a centripetal fashion with a stick with cotton bud, in all four quadrants [47]. The absence of anocutaneous reflex suggests pudendal neuropathy or a cauda equina lesion [48]. ***Digital palpation*** should then be performed gently using a gloved index finger [47]. Anal epithelium and rectal mucosa should be felt for tumor, smoothness, bulging, protruding, and impacted stool. Resting anal sphincter tone and length of anal canal should be noted before asking the patient to squeeze to note voluntary squeeze tone [41, 47]. Then the patient is asked to push and bear down while the examiner places her left hand over the patient's abdomen. The defecation pattern is noted by observing abdominal push effort, anal relaxation, and perineal descent [47]. Patients with suspected pelvic organ prolapse are further examined in a lithotomy position, by asking them to bear down to reveal prolapse of rectum, vaginal, uterus, and/or bladder [41].

By inspection, patients with gaping anus showed lower resting anal sphincter pressure than those without and patients with anal scar had lower incremental squeeze pressure than those without these signs [49]. When comparing squeeze pressure measure by DRE and by high-resolution manometry, there was moderate agreement in the diagnosis of fecal incontinence (ƙ-coefficient = 0.418, p = 0.006).

Sensitivity, specificity, PPV, and NPV were 77.4, 70.0, 88.9, and 50.0%, respectively [50]. Even the agreement is poor if anal resting pressure was used; DRE can be a useful beside test to diagnose FI [50]. Mechanical abnormalities detected during physical examination including palpable mass, mucous bloody stool, and anemia warrant additional investigation such as endoscopy, stool examination, and breath tests [51].

3.2 Anatomical assessment

After secondary FI has been ruled out, investigation to define the underlying mechanism of FI in that patient should be performed. These include endoanal ultrasound or MRI to evaluate anal sphincter and pelvic floor anatomy integrity. For the assessment of anal sphincter defects, DRE is inaccurate for determining external anal sphincter defect <90° (accuracy 36%) [49]. Sensitivity is 90% and specificity is only 27.8% in distinguishing small from extensive anal sphincter defect [52]. Thus, DRE may be able to identify anal sphincter defect but is not sensitive enough to quantify its degree. ***Endoanal ultrasound (EAUS)*** has been recommended as a useful and sensitive tool to detect and define anal sphincter anatomy [44, 45]. It has a firm role in diagnostic work-up of FI [53]. EAUS is the gold standard for morphologic assessment of anal canal [54]. Various kinds of probes are available. Traditional 2D, 360° rotating endoprobe had been used to examine anal canal at multiple levels: (1) uppermost level, U-shaped puborectalis muscle is seen; (2) middle level, complete rings of IAS and EAS were seen and transverse perinei muscle is visualized; and (3) lower level, complete ring of subcutaneous part of EAS was seen without IAS [54, 55]. Normative data using 3D-EAUS had been described in both western and Asian population, and in both genders [56, 57]. Male had longer anal canal length than female by 3D-EAUS [56, 57]; M *vs.* F, 3.9 ± 0.7 *vs.* 3.4 ± 0.43 cm, $p = 0.007$ [57]. Importantly, anterior anal canal length, where puborectalis muscle mass is devoid, is significantly shorter in female [56, 57]; M *vs.* F, 3.6 ± 0.8 vs. 2.8 ± 0.5 cm, $p < 0.001$ [57]. Information which can be obtained included thickness, length, defect, and scar of IAS, EAS components (subcutaneous and superficial parts), and puborectalis muscle. The information of defect and residual anal sphincter remnant can guide anal sphincter repair. **Figure 2** is an example of anal sphincter defect detected by 3D-EAUS. Alternative to EAUS may be transperineal ultrasound (TPUS), which can also detect anal sphincter defect [44]. There was no difference between MRI and EAUS

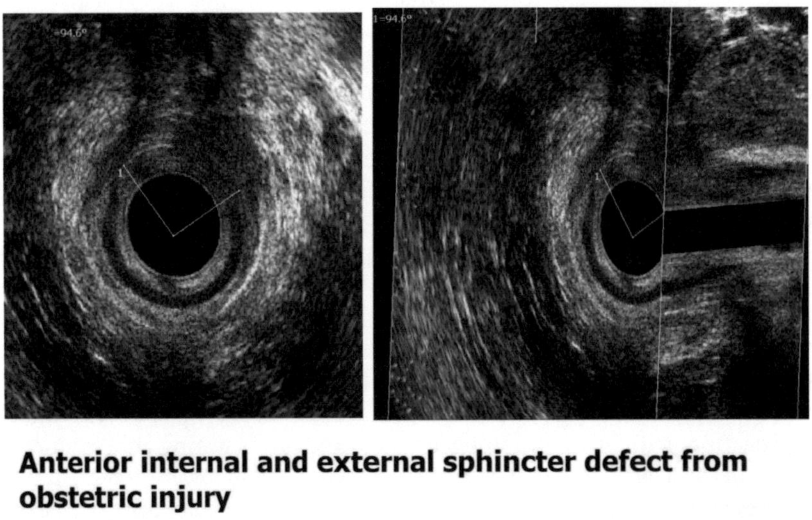

Figure 2.
Anal sphincter defect detected by 3D-endoanal ultrasound.

in depiction of external anal sphincter defect [58]. Sensitivity of MRI vs. EAUS was 81% vs. 90% and the positive predictive value was 89% vs. 85% [58].

In detecting external anal sphincter atrophy, EAUS was also comparable to MRI [59]. External phase-array MRI is comparable to endoanal MRI in detecting EAS atrophy [60]. However, MRI is more expensive and time-consuming than EAUS [45] and is recommended only in the institute with sufficient experience available [60]. Dynamic MRI may be useful in subjects with suspected concomitant pelvic floor disorder, such as rectal prolapse, pelvic organ prolapses, rectocele, enterocele, and perineal descent.

3.3 Functional and neurophysiologic assessment

Anorectal manometry (ARM) has been used to assess global anorectal function. It is used to quantify IAS and EAS function, rectal sensation, rectoanal reflexes, and rectal compliance [51, 61]. Traditional techniques used water-perfused and solid-state probe (6–8 channels). The newer technique uses high-resolution (HRM, 12 channels) and high definition probes (3D-HRM, 256 channels) [51, 61]. From recent international survey, most institutions use a conventional water-perfused system [62]. Solid-state and high-resolution systems are used mostly by specialist center [62]. Techniques and minimum standards of ARM had been described by Rao et al. [63]. These steps can be applied to the new probes. HRM and HDM results were comparable to measurement by water-perfused systems [64, 65]. Important information obtained includes resting anal sphincter pressure which primarily reflects internal anal sphincter function [64, 67]. Resting anal sphincter pressures are varied by gender, age, and testing methodology [28]. Pressure is usually higher in men and younger age [28, 53, 67]. Normal value using classic catheter had been described using solid-state catheter [68]. In our institute, water-perfusion catheter, normative value is shown in **Table 3**. Males had longer high-pressure zone, higher squeeze pressure, and longer squeeze duration than females [68]. **Figure 3** shows manometric findings of a patient with fecal incontinence, in whom, the anal squeeze pressure did not increase as high as normal.

Rectal sensory testing and rectal compliance evaluation can be performed as a part of anorectal manometry or can be performed separately using the barostat technique or electrical stimulus [28]. Incontinent patients may have rectal hyposensitivity or hypersensitivity [51]. Rectal hypersensitivity is commonly found in patients with FI which may be explained by the cognitive precaution of the patients. However, this finding should be studied in detail. Rectal hyposensitivity, found in 10% of subjects with FI, had been reported as a cause of idiopathic FI which may reflect the afferent nerve dysfunction [69, 70]. It may also be due to megarectum and may be associated to fecal retention with overflow FI. Reduced rectal compliance is seen in patients with colitis, low spinal cord lesion, and diabetes mellitus. Increased rectal compliance is seen in high spinal cord lesion [51]. RAIR and cough reflex may be impaired and contribute to FI in some individuals. For example, RAIR may be impaired after low rectal surgery [71] and spinal cord injury below L2 level [72]. Cough reflex is impaired in patients with cauda equina or sacral nerve plexus lesion [28].

Clinical utility of ARM in FI is to assess the weakness of sphincter muscle and abnormal anorectal sensation. For discrimination between normal and incontinent individuals, ARM had reported a sensitivity of 91.4%, an accuracy of 85.8%, and a specificity of 62.5% only [73]. By meta-analysis, ARM is accurate for diagnosis of FI with a sensitivity of 0.80 (95% confidence interval (CI) 0.69–0.88) and a specificity of 0.80 (95%CI 0.65–0.90). The diagnostic likelihood ratio was 16.61 (95%CI 5.52–50.03) [74]. The common parameter used to determine FI was maximal resting pressure [74]. Recent technology of high-definition manometry (HDM) may be able to predict the possibility and to distinguish subjects with FI from healthy subjects [58]. However, further studies are required.

Parameters (mean ± 95%CI)	Male	Female	Total
HPZ rest (cm)	2.4 ± 0.4	2.2 ± 0.2	2.3 ± 0.2
HPZ squeeze (cm)	2.9 ± 0.4	2.8 ± 0.3	2.9 ± 0.3
Resting sphincter pressure (mmHg)	65.3 ± 15.2	58.5 ± 8.3	64.3 ± 8.3
Sustained squeeze pressure (mmHg)	126.9 ± 25.9	102.8 ± 10.3	121.3 ± 14.0
Maximal squeeze pressure (mmHg)	205.8 ± 43.2	169.1 ± 19.1	203.5 ± 23.1
Duration of squeeze (s)	31.8 ± 3.6	29.4 ± 3.1	31.1 ± 2.3
Rectal sensory testing			
Mean first sensation (ml)	15.0 ± 4.3	13.9 ± 3.1	15.1 ± 2.7
Volume at desire to defecate (ml)	35.8 ± 9.5	36.5 ± 6.0	38.7 ± 5.7
Volume at urge to defecate (ml)	61.7 ± 13.8	60.0 ± 8.0	63.8 ± 8.0
Volume at maximal toleration (ml)	120.0 ± 34.1	103.2 ± 16.4	119.1 ± 18.7
Saline continence test			
Saline volume retained (ml)	655.8 ± 72.6	633.2 ± 56.7	638.0 ± 46.0
Mean %volume retained (ml)	90.8 ± 9.3	88.3 ± 7.4	90.0 ± 5.9
Volume at first leak (ml)	313.0 ± 76.4	263.6 ± 52.3	283.1 ± 43.5
Median volume at first leak (ml)	325	280	280
Median retained volume (ml)	750	750	750
Mean % retained volume	100	100	100

**Author's unpublished data.*

Table 3.
*Normative anorectal manometric data.**

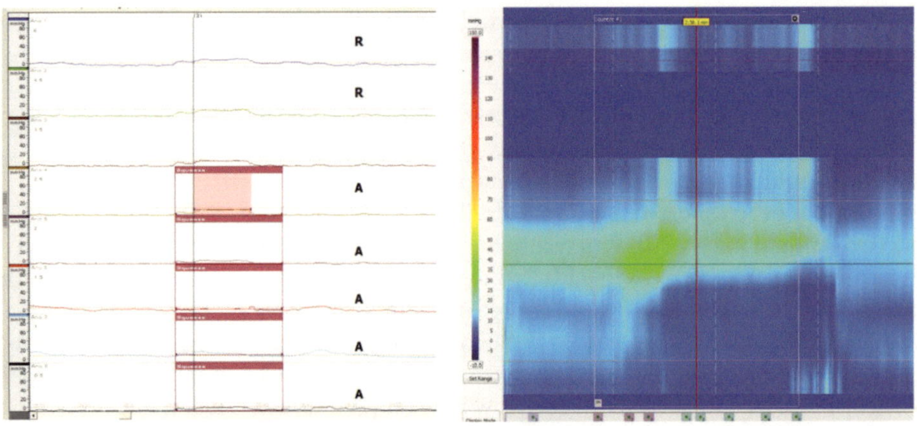

Left: water-perfusion manometric appearance during squeeze; minimal rise in anal sphincter pressure is observed. R-intrarectal pressure, A-intraanal pressure

Right: high-resolution manometric appearance during squeeze; minimal rise of in anal sphincter pressure is observed (note the color reference)

Figure 3.
Anorectal manometric findings in subjects with fecal incontinence during squeeze captured by different techniques; water-perfusion system on the left and high-resolution manometry on the right.

Adjunctive test in FI is the ***saline continence test***, which is performed by infusing 800 ml of 0.9% sodium chloride into the patient's rectum while sitting on a commode at a rate of 60 ml/min [55]. Volume infused at the onset of first leak was about

770 (735–805) ml in male and 530 ml in female (410–650) [68]. The total volume that a male could retain was about 790 (770–810) ml and for a female was 670 (620–750) ml [68]. Subjects with FI had significantly lower volume infused at first leak and total volume retained compared to healthy volunteers [75].

Electromyography (EMG) performed by inserting a needle electrode in the external anal sphincter muscle and levator ani muscle had been used to assess integrity of neuromuscular connection of the muscle [76]. Due to invasiveness, surface EMG had also been used [77]. However, the detection of the EAS defect has been replaced by other imaging techniques such as EAUS and MRI [78], and EMG could not predict the response to biofeedback therapy in FI [79].

Pudendal nerve terminal motor latency test (PNTML) assesses the neuromuscular circuit between the terminal branch of the pudendal nerve and the external anal sphincter by measuring the conduction time between the initial stimulation and the EAS contraction (seen by motor evoked potential curve). Prolonged latency time suggests pudendal neuropathy [76]. However, the test is not sensitive enough to be related with clinical symptoms, manometric findings, and histologic findings [76, 80]. This is because a single intact nerve fiber in a FI patient can give the normal latency time. Thus, it is not routinely recommended [45]. However, in clinical practice, it can be used in conjunction with anorectal manometry and endoanal ultrasound to provide the "missing link" [81] or the possible explanation of underlying pathophysiology of FI in the patient. **Figure 4** demonstrates the abnormal PNTML in a FI patient compared to a normal subject.

Novel neurophysiological investigations can be used to assess the spino-anorectal neuropathy with higher sensitivity. These include ***translumbar and trassacral magnetic neurostimulation*** (***TLMS, TSMS***), which induce motor evoked potential in the anal and rectal areas by using magnetic stimulation at the lumbar and sacral levels [82]. The magnetic stimulation induces the electrical current in the lumbosacral motor nerve roots and then the conduct along the peripheral nerves. The test could detect more anorectal neuropathy than PNTML, is well-tolerated, and can be used to assess the lumbosacral neuropathy in spinal cord injury subjects with anorectal problems [83]. Underlying pathophysiology of fecal incontinence which involves brain-gut axis connection can be tested bi-directionally [84]. For testing efferent pathways, cortical stimulation using transcranial magnetic stimulation over the paramedian motor cortex can be performed [84] and motor-evoked potentials are registered intraluminal at the rectum and anal canal levels. The test has been validated for reproducibility and good interobserver agreement [84]. In one study where both cortico-anorectal and spino-anorectal magnetic stimulations were performed, the peripheral spino-anal and spino-rectal neuropathy was identified to

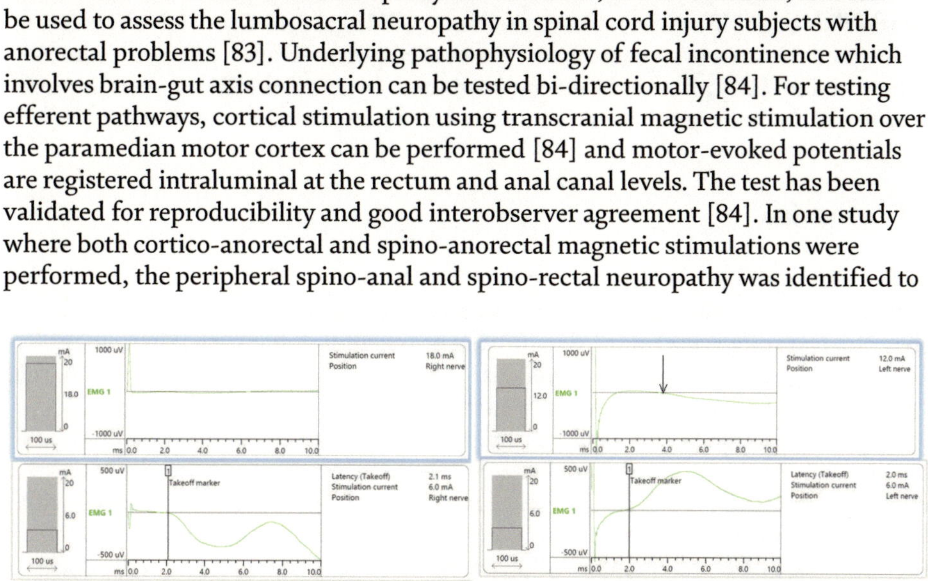

Pudendal Nerve Terminal Motor Latency of subjects with fecal incontinence (upper, blue border) and healthy subjects (lower). In normal subjects latency time was <2.2 msec and in subjects with fecal incontinence the motor evoked potential is not seen on the right and seen with lower amplitude on the left with latency time of about 4.0 msec (arrow)

Figure 4.
Pudendal nerve terminal motor latency testing.

have a possible role in the pathogenesis of FI [85]. For afferent pathways, the cortical sensory perception of anal and rectal stimulation can be detected for cortical evoked potentials (CEPs) using the scalp electrodes [84]. After rectal balloon distension, the prolonged CEP latency was seen in subjects with idiopathic FI [86] suggesting afferent dysfunctions [86]. Brain response to rectal distension can also be detected by functional MRI [28]. Preliminary findings suggested that central cerebral processing of rectal and anal stimuli plays a role in the pathogenesis of FI [29, 86].

3.4 Clinical utility of anorectal anatomical and neurophysiologic tests

FI usually has multiple etiologies including structural and functional defects. Endoanal ultrasound is strongly recommended to detect anal sphincter defects in patients with FI [44, 45]. Three-dimensional ultrasonography is useful to document anal sphincter defects, levator ani muscle avulsion, and tears [44]. Anorectal physiologic tests are used to confirm the diagnosis of FI, to grade the severity, and to determine the underlying pathophysiology. Thus, appropriate management can be planned accordingly. Anorectal manometry provides the baseline resting function of anal sphincter and squeeze function during voluntary contraction. Subjects with FI had shorter high-pressure zone, lower resting, and lower squeeze pressure than normal healthy subjects [75]. In subjects with dyssynergic defecation with overflow continence, the dyssynergic defecation pattern can also be demonstrated [66]. Abnormal anorectal reflex can be demonstrated together with rectal sensation. This information can guide in the biofeedback treatment and planning additional investigation or treatment.

The EMG technique is used to define an underlying neuromuscular dysfunction in selected cases. It is recommended for specialist use in the research study but not in routine clinical practice [28]. PNTML may be useful for assessment of FI especially when considering surgical intervention [28]. The test should be carefully performed and interpreted with caution in conjunction with other investigation results. Other neurophysiologic tests including motor evoked potential after lumbosacral (TLMS, TSMS) and cortical stimulation (TMS) are used to study the efferent brain-gut axis pathways, whereas cortical evoked potential after anorectal stimulation is used to study afferent brain-gut pathways. Functional MRI is a research tool to examine the brain-gut interaction and has not been tested for clinical use [28].

4. Conclusion

Fecal incontinence is a distressing condition of multifactorial etiologies. Detailed clinical evaluation together with selective use of anatomical and neurophysiologic testing is useful for clarification of the underlying pathophysiology. Recent change in bowel habit or stool characters should prompt the attention to rule out secondary FI from organic causes, such as colorectal cancer and inflammatory bowel disease. Severity and quality of life should be assessed. Clinical examination can detect gross, but not minor, defects. 3D-EAUS is recommended to objectively verify anal sphincter integrity. However, anal sphincter scar is better detected with MRI. Dynamic MRI can demonstrate concomitant pelvic floor disorders. TPUS is an alternative to EAUS and dynamic MRI but the accuracy is dependent on the operator's experience. ARM-quantified anal sphincter function measures rectal sensation and compliance. The saline continence test quantifies the severity of FI. EMG has limited clinical utilities and had been replaced by EAUS in detecting the anal sphincter defect. PNTML is insensitive to detect minor neuropathy. TLMS and TSMS are more sensitive to assess the spino-anorectal efferent pathways and TMS assesses the cortico-anorectal efferent pathway. CEP and functional MRI are used to assess the anorectal-cortical afferent pathways. The latter tests for brain-gut-axis are mostly performed in the tertiary specialized institutes. By integration of the patient's all information, management can be planned accordingly. Further study regarding brain-gut-microbiota interaction is continuing for a better understanding of this group of patients.

Conflict of interest

The author has no conflict of interest.

Abbreviations

FI	fecal incontinence
IAS	internal anal sphincter
EAS	external anal sphincter
RAIR	rectoanal inhibitory reflex
CNS	central nervous system
DRE	digital rectal examination
PPV	positive predictive value
NPV	negative predictive value
EAUS	endoanal ultrasound
TPUS	transperineal ultrasound
MRI	magnetic resonance imaging
ARM	anorectal manometry
HRM	high-resolution manometry
CI	confidence interval
HDM	high-definition manometry
EMG	electromyography
PNTML	pudendal nerve terminal motor latency
TLMS	translumbar magnetic stimulation
TSMS	transsacral magnetic stimulation
CEP	cortical evoked potentials
TMS	transcranial magnetic stimulation

Author details

Kasaya Tantiphlachiva
Department of Surgery, Faculty of Medicine, Chulalongkorn University, Bangkok, Thailand

*Address all correspondence to: kasaya.tan@gmail.com

References

[1] Rao SS, Bharucha AE, Chiarioni G, Felt-Bersma R, Knowles C, Malcolm A, et al. Anorectal disorders. Gastroenterology. 2016;**150**:1430-1442

[2] Bedard K, Heyman S, Palsson OS, Bharucha AE, Whitehead WE. Relationship between symptoms and quality of life in fecal incontinence. Neurogastroenterology and Motility. 2018;**30**:313241

[3] McKenna C, Bartlett L, Ho YH. Fecal incontinence reduces quality of life more than you may think. Diseases of the Colon and Rectum. 2017;**60**:e597-e598

[4] Xu X, Menees SB, Zochowski M, Fenner DE. Economic cost of fecal incontinence. Diseases of the Colon and Rectum. 2012;**55**:586-598

[5] Finne-Soveri H, Sørbye LW, Jonsson PV, Carpenter GI, Bernabei R. Increased work-load associated with faecal incontinence among home care patients in 11 European countries. European Journal of Public Health. 2008;**18**:323-328

[6] Macmillan AK, Merrie AE, Marshall RJ, Parry BR. The prevalence of fecal incontinence in community-dwelling adults: A systematic review of the literature. Diseases of the Colon and Rectum. 2004;**47**:1341-1349

[7] Ng KS, Sivakumaran Y, Nassar N, Gladman MA. Fecal incontinence: Community prevalence and associated factors—A systematic review. Diseases of the Colon and Rectum. 2015;**58**:1194-1209

[8] Walter S, Hallbook O, Gotthard R, Bergmark M, Sjodahl R. A population-based study on bowel habits in Swedish community: Prevalence of faecal incontinence and constipation. Scandinavian Journal of Gastroenterology. 2002;**37**:911-916

[9] Demir N, Yuruyen M, Atay K, Yavuzer H, Hatemi I, Doventas A, et al. Prevalence of fecal incontinence and associated risk factors in elderly outpatients: A cross-sectional study. Aging Clinical and Experimental Research. 2017;**29**:1165-1171

[10] Kang HW, Jung HK, Kwon KJ, Song EM, Choi JY, Kim SE, et al. Prevalence and predictive factors of fecal continence. Journal of Neurogastroenterology and Motility. 2012;**18**:86-93

[11] Borrie MJ, Davidson HA. Incontinence in institutions: Costs and contributing factors. Canadian Medical Association Journal. 1992;**147**:322-328

[12] Ihnat P, Kozakova R, Rudinska LI, Peteja M, Vavra P, Zonca P. Fecal incontinence among nursing home residents: Is it still a problem? Archives of Gerontology and Geriatrics. 2016;**65**:79-84

[13] Townsend DC, Carrington EV, Grssi U, Burgell RE, Wong JY, Knowles CH, et al. Pathophysiology of fecal incontinence differs between men and women: A case-matches study in 200 patients. Neurogastroenterology and Motility. 2016;**28**:1580-1588

[14] Guise JM, Morris C, Osterweil P, Li H, Rosenberg D, Greenlick M. Incidence of fecal incontinence after childbirth. Obstetrics and Gynecology. 2007;**109**:281-288

[15] Guillaume A, Salem AE, Garcia P, Chander Roland B. Pathophysiology and therapeutic options for fecal incontinence. Journal of Clinical Gastroenterology. 2017;**51**:324-330

[16] Barucha AE, Blandon RE. Anatomy and physiology of continence. In: Ratto C, Doglietto G, editors. Fecal Incontinence: Diagnosis and Treatment. Milan: Springer; 2007. pp. 3-12

[17] Karpathiotakis M. Pelvic floor anatomy. In: Mongardini M, Giofre M, editors. Management of Fecal Incontinence. Rome: Springer Nature; 2016. pp. 1-9

[18] Kumar L, Emmanuel A. Internal anal sphincter: Clinical perspective. The Surgeon. 2017;**14**:211-226

[19] Nivatvongs S, Gordon PH, Beck D. Surgical anatomy of the colon, rectum and anus. In: Beck D, Wexner S, Rafferty JF, editors. Gordon and Nivatvongs' Principles and Practice of Surgery for the Colon, Rectum and Anus. New York, USA: Thieme Verlagsgruppe; 2019. pp. 1-25

[20] Shafik A. A concept of the anatomy of the anal sphincter mechanism and the physiology of defecation. Diseases of the Colon and Rectum. 1987;**50**:970-982

[21] Gagnard C, Godlewski G, Prat D, Lan O, Cousineau J, Maklouf Y. The nerve branches to the external anal sphincter: The macroscopic supply and microscopic structure. Surgical and Radiologic Anatomy. 1986;**8**:115-119

[22] Yu SW, Rao SS. Anorectal physiologic and pathophysiology in the elderly. Clinics in Geriatric Medicine. 2014;**30**:95-106

[23] Azpiroz F, Fernandez-Fraga X, Merletti R, Enck P. The puborectalis muscle. Neurogastroenterology and Motility. 2005;**17**(Suppl 1):68-72

[24] Bullard Dunn KM, Rothenberger DA. Colon, rectum, and anus. In: Brunicardi F, Andersen DK, Billiar TR, Dunn DL, Hunter JG, Matthews JB, Pollock RE, editors. Schwartz's Principles of Surgery, 10e. New York, NY: McGraw-Hill; 2015. Available from: http://accessmedicine.mhmedical.com.cuml1.md.chula.ac.th/content.aspx?bookid=980&sectionid=59610871 Accessed January 27, 2019

[25] Van Koughnett JA, da Silva G. Anorectal physiology and testing. Gastroenterology Clinics of North America. 2013;**42**:713-728

[26] Uher EM, Swash M. Sacral reflexes: Physiology and clinical application. Diseases of the Colon and Rectum. 1998;**41**:1165-1177

[27] Rao SS. American College of Gastroenterology Practice Parameters Committee. Diagnosis and management of fecal incontinence. The American Journal of Gastroenterology. 2004;**99**:1585-1604

[28] Remes-Troche JM. Neurophysiological testing in anorectal disorders. Expert Review of Gastroenterology & Hepatology. 2008;**2**:323-335

[29] Mirbagheri N, Hatton S, Ng KS, Lagopoulos J, Gladman MA. Brain responses to mechanical rectal stimulation in patients with faecal incontinence: An fMRI study. Colorectal Disease. 2017;**19**:917-926

[30] Lefaucheur JP. Excitability of the motor cortical representation of the external anal sphincter. Experimental Brain Research. 2005;**160**:268-272

[31] Sultan AH, Nugent K. Pathophysiology and nonsurgical treatment of anal incontinence. BJOG. 2004;**111**(Suppl 1):84-90

[32] Shin GH, Toto EL, Schey R. Pregnancy and postpartum bowel changes: Constipation and fecal incontinence. The American Journal of Gastroenterology. 2015;**110**:521-529

[33] Joris F, Hoesli I, Kind A, Ries JJ, Kavvdias T. Obstetrical and epidemiological factors influence the severity of anal incontinence after obstetric anal sphincter injury. BMC Pregnancy and Childbirth. 2019;**19**:94

[34] Cohan JN, Chou AB, Varma MG. Faecal incontinence in men referred for

specialty care: A cross-sectional study. Colorectal Disease. 2015;**17**:802-809

[35] Pucciani F. Post-surgical fecal incontinence. Updates in Surgery. 2018;**70**:477-484

[36] Ruiz NS, Kaiser AM. Fecal incontinence—Challenges and solutions. World Journal of Gastroenterology. 2017;**23**:11-24

[37] Loganathan A, Schloithe AC, Hutton J, Yeoh EK, Fraser R, Dinning PG, et al. Pudendal nerve injury in men with fecal incontinence after radiotherapy for prostate cancer. Acta Oncologica. 2015;**54**:882-888

[38] Schiano di Visconte M, Santoro GA, Cracco N, Sarzo G, Bellio G, Brunner M, et al. Effective of sacral nerve stimulation in fecal incontinence after multimodal oncologic treatment for pelvic malignancies: A multicenter study with 2-year follow-up. Techniques in Coloproctology. 2018;**22**:97-105

[39] Brochard C, Venara A, Bodere A, Ropert A, Bouguen G, Siproudhis L. Pathophysiology of fecal incontinence in obese patents: A prospective case-matched study of 201 patients. Neurogastroenterology and Motility. 2017;**29**:313051

[40] Ortiz H, De Miguel M, Ciga MA. Clinical assessment of the incontinent patient. In: Ratto C, Doglietto G, editors. Fecal Incontinence: Diagnosis and Treatment. Milan: Springer; 2007. pp. 89-93

[41] Alavi K, Chan S, Wise P, Kaiser AM, Sudan R, Bordeianou L. Fecal incontinence: Etiology, diagnosis and management. Journal of Gastrointestinal Surgery. 2015;**19**:1910-1921

[42] Vaizey CJ, Carapeti E, Cahill JA, Kamm MA. Prospective comparison of faecal incontinence grading systems. Gut. 1999;**44**:77-80

[43] Rusavy Z, Jansova M, Kalis V. Anal incontinence severity assessment tools used worldwide. International Journal of Gynaecology and Obstetrics. 2014;**126**:146-150

[44] Italian Society of Colorectal Surgery (SICCR), Pucciani F, Altomare DF, Dodi G, Falletto E, Frasson A, et al. Diagnosis and treatment of faecal incontinence: Consensus statement of the Italian Society of Colorectal Surgery and the Italian association of hospital gastroenterologists. Digestive and Liver Disease. 2015;**47**:628-645

[45] Paquette IM, Varma MG, Kaiser AM, Steele SR, Rafferty JF. The American Society of Colon and Rectal Surgeons' clinical practice guideline for the treatment of fecal incontinence. Diseases of the Colon and Rectum. 2015;**58**:623-636

[46] Rockwood TH, Church JM, Fleshman JW, Kane RL, Mavran- tonis C, Thorson AG, et al. Fecal incontinence quality of life scale: Quality of life instrument for patients with fecal incontinence. Diseases of the Colon and Rectum. 2000;**43**:9-17

[47] Tantiphlachiva K, Rao P, Attaluri A, Rao SSC. Digital rectal examination is a useful tool for identifying patients with dyssynergia. Clinical Gastroenterology and Hepatology. 2010;**8**:955-960

[48] Andromanakos NP, Filippou DK, Pinis SI, Kostakis AI. Anorectal incontinence: A challenge in diagnostic and therapeutic approach. European Journal of Gastroenterology & Hepatology. 2013;**25**:1247-1256

[49] Dobben AC, Terra MP, Deutekom M, Gerhards MF, Bijnen AB, Felt-Bersma RJ, et al. Anal inspection and digital rectal examination compared to anorectal physiology tests and endoanal ultrasonography in evaluating fecal incontinence. International Journal of Colorectal Disease. 2007;**22**:783-790

[50] Soh JS, Lee HJ, Jung KW, Yoon IJ, Koo HS, Seo SY, et al. The diagnostic value of a digital rectal examination compared with high-resolution anorectal manometry in patients with chronic constipation and fecal incontinence. The American Journal of Gastroenterology. 2015;**110**:1197-1204

[51] Rao SSC. Advances in diagnostic assessment of fecal incontinence and dyssynergic defecation. Clinical Gastroenterology and Hepatology. 2010;**8**:910-919

[52] Coura MM, Silva SM, Almeida RM, Forrest MC, Sousa JB. Is digital rectal exam reliable in grading anal sphincter defectas? Arquivos de Gastroenterologia. 2016;**53**:240-245

[53] Olson CH. Diagnostic testing for fecal incontinence. Clinics in Colon and Rectal Surgery. 2014;**27**:85-90

[54] Abdool Z, Sultan AH, Thakar R. Ultrasound imaging of the anal sphincter complex: A review. The British Journal of Radiology. 2012;**85**:865-875

[55] Stone DE, Quiroz LH. Ultrasound imaging of the pelvic floor. Obstetrics and Gynecology Clinics of North America. 2016;**43**:141-153

[56] Knowles AM, Knowles CH, Scott SM, Lunniss PJ. Effects of age and gender on three-dimensional endoanal ultrasonography measurements: Development of normal ranges. Techniques in Coloproctology. 2008;**12**:323-329

[57] Tantiphlachiva K, Sahakitrungruang C, Pattanaarun J, Rojanasakul A. Normative anatomy of the anal sphincter detected with 3D-endoanal ultrasonography. Asian Biomedicine. 2013;7:865-871

[58] Zifan A, Ledgerwooe-Lee M, Mittal RK. A predictive model to identify patients with fecal incontinence based on high-definition manometry. Clinical Gastroenterology and Hepatology. 2016;**14**:178-196

[59] Cazemier M, Terra MP, Stoker J, de Lange-de Klerk ES, Boeckxstaens GE, Mulder CJ, et al. Atrophy and defects detection of the external anal sphincter: Comparison between three-dimensional anal endosonography and endoanal magnetic resonance imaging. Diseases of the Colon and Rectum. 2006;**49**:20-27

[60] Terra MP, Beets-Tan RG, van der Hulst VP, Deutekom M, Dijkgraaf MG, Bossuyt PM, et al. MRI in evaluating atrophy of the external anal sphincter in patients with fecal incontinence. American Journal of Roentgenology. 2006;**187**:99109

[61] Bharucha AE, Rao SS. An update on anorectal disorders for gastroenterologists. Gastroenterology. 2014;**146**:37-45

[62] Carrington EV, Heinrich H, Knowles CH, Rao SS, Fox M, Scott SM. Methods of anorectal manometry vary widely in clinical practice: Results from an international survey. Neurogastroenterology and Motility. 2017;**29**:e13016. DOI: 10.1111/nmo.13016

[63] Rao SSC, Azpiroz F, Diamant N, Enck P, Tougass G, Wald A. Minimum standards of anorectal manometry. Neurogastroenterology and Motility. 2002;**14**:553-559

[64] Kang HR, Lee JE, Lee JS, Lee TH, Hong SJ, Kim JO, et al. Comparison of high-resolution anorectal manometry with water-perfused anorectal manometry. Journal of Neurogastroenterology and Motility. 2015;**21**:126-132

[65] Vitton V, Ben Hadj Amor W, Baumstarch K Grimaud JC, Bouvier M. Water-perfused manometry vs. three-dimensional high-resolution

manometry: A comparative study on a large patient population with anorectal disorders. Colorectal Disease. 2013;**15**:e726-e731. DOI: 10.1111/codi.12397

[66] Staller K. Role of anorectal manometry in clinical practice. Current Treatment Options in Gastroenterology. 2015;**13**:418-431

[67] Lee HR, Lim SB, Park JY. Anorectal manometric parameters are influenced by gender and age in subjects with normal bowel function. International Journal of Colorectal Disease. 2014;**29**:1393-1399

[68] Rao SS, Hatfield R, Soffer E, Rao S, Beaty J, Conklin JL. Manometric tests of anorectal function in healthy adults. The American Journal of Gastroenterology. 1999;**94**:773-783

[69] Burgell RE. Hyposensitivity SSMR. Journal of Neurogastroenterology and Motility. 2012;**18**:373-384

[70] Madbouly KM, Hussein AM. Temporary sacral nerve stimulation in patients with fecal incontinence owing to rectal hyposensitivity: A prospective, double-blind study. Surgery. 2015;**157**:56-63

[71] Kakodkar R, Gupta S, Nundy S. Low anterior resection with total mesorectal excision for rectal cancer: Functional assessment and factors affecting outcome. Colorectal Disease. 2006;**8**:650-656

[72] Thiruppathy K, Mason J, Akbari K, Raeburn A, Emmanuel A. Physiological study of the anorectal reflex in patients with functional anorectal and defecation disorders. Journal of Digestive Diseases. 2017;**18**:222-228

[73] Pehl C, Seidl H, Scalecio N, Gundling F, Schmidt T, Schepp W, et al. Accuracy of anorectal manometry in patients with fecal incontinence. Digestion. 2012;**86**:78-85

[74] Yeap ZH, SImillis C, Qiu S, Ramage L, Kontovounisios C, Tekkis P. Diagnostic accuracy of anorectal manometry for fecal incontinence: A meta-analysis. Acta Chirurgica Belgica. 2017;**117**:347-355

[75] Tantiphlachiva K, Pattana-arun J, Sahakitrungrueng C, Rojanasakul A. Comprehensive evaluation of fecal incontinence: A preliminary report of anatomical neurophysiology study. Journal of the Medical Association of Thailand. 2018;**101**(Suppl 4):S29-S37

[76] Kumar A, Rao SS. Diagnostic testing in fecal incontinence. Current Gastroenterology Reports. 2003;**5**:406-413

[77] Nowakowski M, Tomaszewski KA, Herman RM, Salowka J, Romaniszyn M, Rubinkiewicz M, et al. Developing a new electromyography-based algorithm to diagnose the etiology of fecal incontinence. International Journal of Colorectal Disease. 2014;**29**:747-754

[78] Dobben AC, Terra MP, Deutekom M, Bossuyt PM, Felt-Bersma RJ, Stoker J. Diagnostic Work-up for Faecal Incontinence in Daily Clinical Practice in the Netherlands

[79] Lacima G, Pera M, Gonzalez-Argente X, Torrents A, Valls-Sole J, Espuna-Pons M. Is electromyography a predictive test of patient response to biofeedback in the treatment of fecal incontinence? Neurourology and Urodynamics. 2016;**35**:390-394

[80] Osterberg A, Graf W, Eeg-Olofsson K, Hynninen P, Pahlman L. Results of neurophysiologic evaluation in fecal incontinence. Diseases of the Colon and Rectum. 2000;**43**:1256-1261

[81] Remes-Troche JM, Rao SSC. Neurophysiological testing in anorectal

disorders. Expert Rev Gasroenterol Hepatol. 2008;**2**:323-335

[82] Rao SSC, Coss-Adame E, Tantiphlachiva K, Attaluri A, Remes-Troche J. Translumbar and transsacral magnetic neuro-stimulation for the assessment of neuropathy in fecal incontinence. Diseases of the Colon and Rectum. 2014;**57**:645-652

[83] Tantiphlachiva K, Attaluri A, Valestin J, Yamada T, Rao SSC. Translumabar and transsacral motor-evoked potentials: A novel test for spino-anorectal neuropathy in spinal cord injury. The American Journal of Gastroenterology. 2011;**106**:907-914

[84] Remes-Troche JM, Tantiphlachiva K, Attaluri A, Valestin J, Yamada T, Hamdy S, et al. A bi-directional assessment of the human brain-anorectal axis. Neurogastroenterology and Motility. 2011;**23**:240-e118. DOI: 10.1111/j.1365-2982.2010.01619.x

[85] Xiang X, Patcharatrakul T, Sharma A, Parr R, Hamdy S, Rao SSO. Cortico-anorecatl, spino-anorectal, and cortico-spinal nerve conduction and locus of neuronal injury in patients with fecal incontinence. Clinical Gastroenterology and Hepatology. 2018. DOI: 10.1016/j.cgh.2018.09.007

[86] Haas S, Brock C, Krogh K, Gram M, Lundby L, Drewes AM, et al. Abnormal neuronal response to rectal and anal stimuli in patients with idiopathic fecal incontinence. Neurogastroenterology and Motility. 2015;**27**:954-962

Chapter 3

Quality of Life Considerations on Fecal Incontinence

Arantxa Muñoz Duyos and Yolanda Ribas

Abstract

Traditionally, it has been assumed that tests like anorectal manometry and endoanal ultrasound are essential in the evaluation of fecal incontinence (FI). However, in daily practice, this testing rarely helps in the decision-making, as are mainly based on the patient's symptoms. Moreover, indications and outcome evaluation should not be decided by only considering the symptom severity but the impact on QoL and patient satisfaction. Nowadays, patients tend to be active consumers of health care, so they may participate on the medical decision-making. On the other hand, monitoring treatment results are mandatory in current practice. Finally, considering the cost of some of the current treatments for FI, changes in QoL should be demonstrated before implementing some procedures. For all these reasons, the QoL scales should be used, and readers encouraged to become familiar with QoL instruments and their limitations. The following chapter will cover almost all areas on existing knowledge about QoL in patients with FI: from how many types of QOL scales have been described, to the different ways to measure our patients' satisfaction, passing through the difference between severity and QOL, going deep on if the improvement of patients treated for FI is reflected enough in the current used QOL scales.

Keywords: Quality of Life, Fecal Incontinence, Evaluation, Severity, Patients' satisfaction

1. Introduction

Quality of life (QoL) is the general well-being of an individual including all the emotional, social and physical aspects. A half century ago, the WHO defined QoL as an "individual's perception of their position in life in the context of the culture and value systems in which they live and in relation to their goals, expectations, standards and concerns" [1]. Therefore, the concept was already multidimensional including physical, mental and social domains. Health-Related Quality of Life (HRQoL) has been defined as the "physical, psychological, and social domains of health, seen as distinct areas that are influenced by a person's experiences, beliefs, expectations and perceptions" [2]. In other words, it would be an assessment of how the individual's well-being may be affected over time by a disease, disability or disorder.

Patients should be actively involved in the treatment decisions, and therefore, the assessment of health perception is essential. Therapeutic outcomes are not meaningful if they are not balanced with the patient's perception of QoL, thus asking patients about their health and QoL before and after a procedure is crucial to improve the quality of care. Patient-reported outcomes are reports coming directly from patients about how they feel or function in relation to a health condition and its treatment without any interpretation by healthcare professionals or anyone else [3].

In the last 30 years, different instruments assessing HRQoL and the broader concept of patient-reported outcomes have been developed. These instruments do not substitute the physical, physiological or biochemical evaluations, as they are complementary and represent the patient's general perception of the effect of illness and treatment in different aspects of life such as physical, psychological and social [4].

Fecal incontinence (FI) is a social and emotionally devastating condition that significantly affects the QoL of patients and their families, and the ultimate goal of treatment should be to improve it, being essential to obtain direct data from the patient. Considering that it is a symptom, the subjective perception is essential in assessing the impact of incontinence on QoL. Patients commonly experience embarrassment, and some people limit their social life to assure an easy access to a toilet. Unfortunately, given the social stigma associated with the condition, many patients do not seek treatment. It has been suggested that the prevalence in the general population has been systematically underestimated, to the point that it has been proposed that healthcare professionals should improve detection by actively enquiring about symptoms of FI in high-risk groups [5]. The fact that only 5–27% of people report their symptoms to their physicians may justify the low number of published studies assessing the QoL in patients with FI [6].

This chapter will cover almost all areas on the existing knowledge about FI patients' QoL.

2. Types of QoL scales

There are two ways of administering questionnaires: by a face-to-face interview or in a self-administered way. Traditionally, face-to face surveys have been considered the gold standard because of their ability to obtain high response rates and valid data. However, in QoL questions, it seems that less bias in responses is produced by self-administered questionnaires due to the embarrassing situation of confessing such sensitive questions to an interviewer [7]. Furthermore, face-to-face surveys are more expensive.

Having an alternative viewpoint on a patient's QOL provided by family caregivers or other proxies is important to avoid excluding patients who cannot respond for themselves due to some cognitive impairment, of in case of very young children. Furthermore, proxy assessment of health utility may also supplement critical information for clinical decision-making on economic evaluations of patients care and health of cost-effectiveness and cost-utility analyses [8]. Proxy-patient agreement is lower for more subjective measures (e.g., expectations and satisfaction with social activities) compared with more objective ones (e.g., the frequency of social participation) [9].

In case of children, parent-proxy rapport can often be a limitation in the assessment of QOL [10], with only a few studies evaluating the level of agreement between parents and children on a child's QOL over time. A large study [11] showed low to moderate levels of parent-child agreement at baseline and lower agreement at follow-up; child's age and parent's self-perceived health were the primary factors associated with parent-child disagreements over time. Based on these findings, authors recommended direct self-assessment of QOL among children and adolescents as much as possible.

Most QoL questionnaires are self-administered and they take into account both the physical and the emotional aspects, which are usually divided in different dimensions, the domains.

For the development of a questionnaire, several questions have to be considered:

1. *Validity*: it is the degree to which evidence and theory support the interpretations of test scores entailed by the proposed uses of tests [12]. Validity refers to whether the questionnaire actually measures what it is intended to measure and not something else, so it has to be established whether the questions and the responses are phrased appropriately. Thus, it has to be determined how representative the questions are (content validity), an association between the test scores and the prediction of a theoretical trait has to be demonstrated (construct validity), and if the questionnaire is measuring what it is intended to measure (criterion validity).

2. *Reliability*: it is the ability of the questionnaire to yield reproducible and consistent estimates of true treatment effect [12]. Reliability means that the responses to the questionnaire are reproducible and that it has internal consistency as well.

3. *Responsiveness*: the instrument should be able to detect the changes in the expected outcomes. For instance, if a questionnaire is determining the QoL of certain condition, then it should be able to predict the QoL after treating that condition.

Furthermore, in order to avoid erroneous research conclusions, the translation of questionnaires should undergo an appropriate and rigorous validation process, as it was done by the International Quality of Life Assessment (IQOLA) project to translate the S-36 Health Survey [13]. Questionnaires must adapt in a culturally relevant and comprehensible form while keeping the original meaning and intention [13, 14].

Studies assessing the QoL in patients with FI have used three types of questionnaires: generic QoL scales, specialized scales and condition-specific scales.

Generic QoL Scales try to cover all aspects of life and are summarized in an overall score. They are commonly used to measure QoL in patients with more than one disease, and they permit comparison of QoL across groups of patients with different medical conditions. Generic scales enable researchers to look at the target population relative to other populations. They are usually adequate for detecting gross changes in a specific population, but they often lack the specific questions to detect subtle changes and, in the case of FI, many remarkable aspects may not be reflected. For FI, the most widely used generic questionnaire is the Short Form 36 Health Status Questionnaire (SF-36) [15].

Specialized scales have been developed for a specific condition or symptom, not a specific population. These scales focus on the measurement of a particular aspect of QoL, such as the assessment of sleeping disorders in patients with irritable bowel syndrome [16] or depression in patients with FI [17]. Specialized scales provide two advantages. First, there is a lower probability that other dimensions of life will emerge, and the instrument will therefore probably be more responsive to change. Second, as with general QoL measures, specialized scales allow for comparison across different populations (for instance, comparing the presence of depression in FI versus depression in multiple sclerosis). The main disadvantage of specialized scales is that the global sense of QoL is not reflected [18].

Condition-specific scales are specially designed to go deep into QoL aspects in each group of patients and its main advantage is that they can be used to detect changes in the treated population. However, as expected, these instruments cannot be used to compare QoL between different diseases. Four different types of condition-specific scales have been used to assess QoL in FI, each of them with strengths and weaknesses that will be further explained. The first one, the Fecal Incontinence Quality of Life Scale (FIQL), has been used as an evaluation tool for patients with FI and it has been widely translated [19]. The second one, the Gastrointestinal Quality of Life Index (GIQLI) [20], is an instrument for measuring QoL specifically in patients with gastrointestinal disorders, which has the additional advantage of looking at FI relative to other gastrointestinal diseases. Finally, the third type would be condition-specific quality instruments, which are designed to assess QoL in specific populations. The Manchester Health Questionnaire (MHQ) [21] was adapted to measure the condition-specific QoL related to FI from a validated measure of urinary incontinence (the King's Health Questionnaire [22]). Subsequently, the Modified Manchester Health Questionnaire (MMHQ) [23] was developed by combining the Fecal Incontinence Severity Scale (FISI) and the MHQ.

3. Measuring the impact of FI: the difference between severity and QoL

Initial scores to assess FI did not include questions about QoL [24, 25]. The most frequently used questionnaires, the Cleveland Clinic Continence Score (CCCS) [26] and the St Mark's score [27], have demonstrated and excellent intra and interobserver reliability [28] and they added a question about lifestyle alterations, with answers ranking in time frequency. However, ranking limitations in daily activities on the basis of time frequency may be difficult for patients. Furthermore, a person who has adapted oneself to deal with episodes of FI over a long period of time may not realize the magnitude of the impact that these episodes have been having on the activities of daily living.

Moreover, severity scores in FI were developed to be as objective as possible but introducing variables such as coping mechanisms and lifestyle changes tends to add subjective aspects, thus they should be interpreted with caution [29].

Additionally, some limitations in applying some scores should be mentioned. Both the CCCS and the St Mark's score characterize the frequency of each type of incontinence separately (i.e. solid, liquid or gas). However, other authors consider that it is difficult for patients to specify and, consequently, their scale has been developed using a different grading system, as in the Fecal Incontinence and Constipation Assessment (FICA) scale [30].

Moreover, health professionals have an additional difficulty scoring the frequency of liquid stool incontinence. In patients never experiencing liquid stools, score could be considered both in the CCCS and the St Mark's score, but if the question is what patient think that it would happen in case that they had liquid stools, score could be 4.

Other significant limitations when assessing FI are: (a) most scores do not include urgency, with the exception of the FICA and the St Mark's score and (b) the FICA score is the only one that quantifies the amount of leakage, thus in other questionnaires the severity of FI would be identical for a minor staining or a large bowel leakage once a week [31].

For all the reasons mentioned above, we need to be aware that severity alone may not be sufficient to establish a therapeutic decision.

As a result, some authors have tried to correlate the QoL assessments with the severity scores. Eypasch et al. [20] determined that patients with a CCCS over 9 had a severe alteration in their QoL measured by the Gastrointestinal Quality of Life Índex (GIQLI), and that they rested home with very poor social activities.

Bharucha et al. correlated the FICA symptom severity score and a modification of the FIQL scale, and concluded that the FICA score is a simple instrument to use in the office, and that it demonstrates reasonably both the physical manifestations of FI (i.e. symptom severity) but also the impact on QOL [31].

However, the correlation between severity and QoL questionnaires is still a controversial issue. Impact on QoL varies between patients depending on daily activity, work, personality and many other dimensions. While one episode of solid FI might represent a significant trauma leading to changes in personal and working life for one patient, another one might consider it significant just in the case that it happened frequently. Consequently, gas incontinence may be a significant problem for a young person with an active social and working life, but it may not be considered as important for other people.

Rockwood et al. reported that patients acknowledged gas incontinence being more severe than what their doctors considered, being the opposite regarding solid FI [19]. This difference is due to the fact that severity scores are constructed under a pathophysiologic point of view mainly reflecting the doctor's perspective. Thus, gas incontinence is considered less severe by doctors, as they don't expect to find a significant structural or functional disorder when compared with a patient with solid stool incontinence.

Furthermore, FI assessment of the outcome of treatments for FI measurement should take into account the impact on lifestyle. For instance, improving gas incontinence in a young person with an active working life, could decrease the severity score less than 20%, but, however, have a significant impact on QoL.

4. Measuring QoL in fecal incontinence

The Short Form-36 (SF-36) is a multidimensional questionnaire constructed to survey health status in the Medical Outcomes Study [15]. It is used in clinical practice and research, as well as health policy evaluations and general population surveys.

The questionnaire includes 36 items grouped in 8 dimensions: limitations in physical activities, limitations in social activities, limitations in usual role activities because of physical health problems, bodily pain, general mental health, limitations in usual role activities because of emotional problems, vitality (energy and fatigue) and general health perceptions. The SF-36 is scaled from 0 to 100, where higher scores represent a better health status. The questionnaire was designed for self-administration as well as for administration by a trained interviewer either by telephone or in person. The questionnaire has been sufficiently validated and its main advantage is that it is easy and relatively fast to fill in, taking 10–20 minutes as an average. It is the most used instrument to validate other questionnaires subsequently designed and to assess the specific questionnaires.

The SF-36 allows us to compare FI populations with urinary incontinence patients or to compare FI populations with altogether different populations, such as healthy persons or persons with other chronic diseases [13].

As other generic scales, the main disadvantage of the SF-36 is that while the "role physical" measurement might be sufficient to detect changes among persons with FI, the "role social" measurement is probably not sensitive enough to detect such changes (i.e. going to a movie or travelling) [32].

The Gastrointestinal Quality of Life Index (GIQLI) [15] is a "systemic", but not generic, QoL instrument designed to be administered across all populations with gastrointestinal conditions, which has also been used to assess FI. The questionnaire was designed in three phases and it was also validated against other generic measures of QoL. The GIQLI contains 36 questions, each with 5 response categories, in 5 areas: a symptom list, physical issues (function and perception of functional ability), psychological issues (primarily affect), social issues and disease-specific items (items tied directly to a specific condition, such as bowel urgency for FI). The significant advantage of this type of instrument over condition-specific QoL measures is its ability to look at FI relative to other gastrointestinal conditions [18].

The FIQL scale is the most widely used condition specific QoL instrument in FI. It was developed by a panel of experts, including colorectal surgeons and health service researchers, that selected aspects (or domains) of QoL likely to be affected by FI [19, 33]. The study included 190 participants (118 patients with FI and 72 controls) from 5 different clinics. The psychometric evaluation showed that the questionnaire produced a reliable and valid measurement of QoL in patients with FI. The questionnaire is self-administered, and it includes questions regarding the limitations in their activities caused by FI during the last month.

The FIQL scale includes 29 items that are grouped into 4 scales or domains:

- Lifestyle: comprising 10 questions about the limitation in social activities such as dining out, travelling, or even basic activities such as shopping.

- Coping/behaviour: including 9 questions relating to the level of concern of FI in daily thoughts, and the limitation that represents on sexual relations, work, etc.

- Depression/self-perception: comprising 7 questions about the impact of FI on their feelings, and how they see themselves in their environment.

- Embarrassment and feeling of social rejection, including 3 questions.

Possible answers range from 1 to 4, where 1 indicates a low functional status. The score of each domain is obtained from the mean of all items. The scale includes a "not applicable" category that is coded as a null value in the final sum, although the author recommends not to use it as a response option [33]. Thus, the four domains are scored from 1 to 4, and the higher score better QoL.

The main advantages of the FIQL scale are that it can be used in all adult populations with FI regardless their particular characteristics, and that it is sensitive to the dynamic relationship between the condition, the treatment, and QoL. A recent study re-evaluated the FIQL and confirmed several strengths but also has pointed out some limitations warranting a revision [34].

The Manchester Health Questionnaire (MHQ) [21] was made up of items adapted from the King's Health Questionnaire [22], a condition-specific HRQOL to evaluate urinary incontinence. The MHQ contains 31 items that are grouped into 9 subscales: general health, physical limitations, social function, role limitations, emotional problems, sexual function, sleep/energy, incontinence impact and incontinence severity. Scores range between 0 and 100, a higher score indicating impairment of HRQOL. The questionnaire was evaluated for content validity by 15 females with known FI, and pre-tested for ambiguity and ease of comprehension in a group of 15 females without known FI and in 20 midwives. Interestingly, during pre-testing, it was found that women had difficulty understanding words such as "fecal" and "stool" and thus, wording was replaced with the term "bowel leakage." The final questionnaire showed excellent internal consistency, test-retest reliability, criterion validity and construct validity.

Scores on the MHQ were compared with scores on the SF-36 reaching modest to strong correlations depending on the domain, but the pattern of correlation between the individual scales of the measures was not specified.

As the instrument appeared promising, it has been suggested that further research is required to validate the measure and test sensitivity to change, before it could be used as a primary end point for studies. Moreover, research comparing the MHQ and the FIQL scale would be also useful as the sampled content is similar [32].

The Modified Manchester Health Questionnaire (MMHQ) [23] is a telephone-administered version of the Fecal Incontinence Severity Scale (FISI) [29] and the Manchester Health Questionnaire [21]. Questions from the FISI were combined with similar questions from the MHQ, and some of the MHQ questions, which had been validated in the UK, were rephrased to make them more consistent with American English. Although the authors planned to collect data from 50 female patients, they achieved a relatively small sample as only 30 patients provided data, being incomplete in 4 of them. The MMHQ includes 8 subscales: overall impact, role limitations, physical/social limitations, personal relationships, emotions, sleep/energy, sexual activity and lifestyle adaptation. The MMHQ is scaled from 0 to 100, for total and subscale scores, where higher scores represent a negative impact on HRQOL. In an invited commentary in the same article, Rockwood considered that whether the MMHQ is a viable instrument for a telephone assessment of QoL in FI remains to be established due to the risk of measurement error [23].

The International Consultation on Incontinence Questionnaire–Bowel Symptoms (ICIQ-B) [35] was developed by a multidisciplinary team of clinical experts in order to evaluate symptoms of FI and impact on HRQOL in a general adult population. The goal was to design an instrument including the patient's input that could be used globally in clinical practice or research. The ICIQ-B has 21 items evaluating bowel pattern, bowel control and HRQOL. Scores are generated for each section; the higher the score, the greater the symptom severity and bother to the patient. The instrument has undergone psychometric evaluation and deemed to be valid, reliable and responsive, and it is well suited to clinical practice. The questionnaire also queries the patient to rank issues that are most bothersome.

There are other types of impact measures less frequently used that need to be mentioned. Although further investigation is required, they might prove to be useful tools in the future.

The TyPE specification designed by Wexner and colleagues [36] was developed to measure the fear of incontinence and how activities were affected by using a single question: "During the past 4 weeks, did fear of bowel accidents or leakage limit your participation in the following activities?". Listed activities are: walking, vigorous exercise, household chores, visiting friends, driving, sexual relations, employment, traveling, church or temple attendance and shopping. There are no summary scores for the measure, and thus, each item is evaluated individually. Very little information is available about the development of the measure and information on reliability is not available.

The Direct Questionning of Objectives (DQO) measure consists of a highly personal assessment, constructed on the basis of each patient's feelings. To calculate the DQO, patients list different objectives that are important for them, such as travelling or working, rate the importance of each objective on a scale and also rate their ability to perform that objective in another scale, both from 0 to 10. The product of ability and performance for each objective is calculated and divided by 10. This number is added for all objectives and divided by the importance scores for all objectives, resulting in a score from 0 to 1.0. The main disadvantages of this system of ranking the impact are: (a) the initial generation of objectives and importance ratings require assistance by trained personnel; (b) it is a cognitively more complex task than completing a questionnaire and (c) measuring only certain individualized objectives may decrease the validity of the measure when groups of patients are to be compared. However, on the other side, the result is directly relevant to a specific person, so it would be more useful when deciding the treatment of an individual patient. This measure has been used to assess the QoL in patients on home parenteral nutrition after surgery for inflammatory bowel disease and also to assess the impact of neuropathic FI on QoL [37].

A study [38] analyzing the validation of QoL measures in FI concluded that the scales with the strongest degree of validity are the GIQLI, FIQL and the ICIQ-B although all of them have some deficiency. The FIQL is the most widely used by far, the main reason for this probably being that it was constructed on a strong methodological basis, being useful and sensitive to change. However, there may be other factors such as habit and the easiness to use it, as it has fewer domains than other questionnaires. Furthermore, the FIQL scale has been translated into many languages (French, Portuguese, Italian, Spanish, Turkish, German, Norwegian and Japanese).

5. What do we know about QoL in patients with FI?

Over the last 25 years, there have been improvements in the understanding, diagnosis and treatment of FI. Although FI has a major impact on QoL, it was not discussed in the literature until 15 years ago.

Few studies in elderly patients showed alterations in specific domains of the SF-36 questionnaire, such as the emotional role, mental health and physical role [39, 40]. However, in younger populations, the assessment of the impact of FI on QoL including specific questions such as change in eating patterns, work, social and sexual activities, only began when disease-specific measures were designed (**Table 1**).

Initially, aspects concerning QoL came from epidemiological studies performed in the general population. Perry and colleagues [41] designed a population-based study using a postal questionnaire that was mailed to almost 16,000 subjects aged 40 years or more. Although it was published in 2002, the study was designed before the development of the FIQL scale, and QoL was measured using general questions: Do your bowel symptoms: bother you?; cause you any physical discomfort?; interfere with your daily activities?, interfere with your social life?; affect your relationships with other people?, upset or distress you?, affect your sleep? and affect your overall QoL? Overall, the prevalence of at least a monthly leakage was 3.3% and the prevalence of soiling was 2.7%. Half of the patients with major FI and, interestingly, 16% of patients with minor FI reported that their bowel symptoms had a significant impact on their life. Nearly two thirds of this group reported to need help for their symptoms.

A panel of experts including colorectal surgeons and health service researchers, was invited to identify QOL-related domains adversely affected by FI, leading to the development of the FIQL scale [19]. An extensive research in two distinct populations demonstrated that patients with FI had a significantly lower QoL than the control population (patients with other gastrointestinal problems). The study demonstrated that these patients reduce activities that other people take for granted such as shopping, going to the cinema, dining out or having sexual intercourse. They suffer from embarrassment, shame and sometimes depression. This was the first evidence that specific daily activities are affected in patients with FI.

Author	Year	N	Population studied	Questionnaires	QoL alterations
O'Keefe et al. [39], Edwards and Jones [40]	1995 2001	704 2818	Elderly patients	SF-36	-Emotional role, mental health, and physical role
Perry et al. [41]	2002	16.000	Population-based study, >40 years old Postal questionnaire	Specific questions "Do your bowel symptoms:....?"	–50% with major FI and 16% with minor FI reported that bowel symptoms had a negative impact on their life -Nearly two thirds of this group said they wanted help with symptoms
Rockwood et al. [29]	2000	190	FI vs. other gastrointestinal disorders	FIQL	-FI patients reduced shopping, going to the cinema, dining out or having sexual intercourse -FI patients suffer from embarrassment, shame and sometimes depression
Bordeianou et al. [42]	2008	502	Patients referred to a Pelvic Floor Centre because of FI	FIQL + SF-36	-All domains of FIQL significantly altered -Coping-behaviour and embarrassment the two most affected -SF-36 scores decreased as the severity of FI increased, with the exception of the scales on pain, physical role and physical functioning -FI patients were worse than those with rheumatoid arthritis or diabetes, and as severely affected as patients with inflammatory bowel disease
Bharucha et al. [30]	2006	2800	Population-based study Postal questionnaire	FIQL adaptation FICA score	-Urgency affect more QoL -<1 episode/month had important impact on QoL -More affected activities in which toilet access was unpredictable or activities that involved eating

Author	Year	N	Population studied	Questionnaires	QoL alterations
Boreham et al. [43]	2005	457	Women presenting for gynecologic care	FIQL FISI	-Embarrassment the most affected domain -Almost 50% thought that there was no treatment available -Few of them had previously sought care
Bartlett et al. [44]	2009	154	Patients attending a urogynecology and colorrectal clinic for other conditions	FIQL	-QoL severely affected by FI in all four scales -Increased bowel frequency, quantity of fecal loss, type of incontinence and fecal urgency -No difference in QOL when comparing weekly and monthly incontinent episodes
Markland et al. [45]	2010	155	Women presenting with FI in a specialty clinic	MMHQ FISI	-Younger women had worst QoL -Increased bowel movement frequency and urgency worst QoL -Urinary incontinence, prior cholecystectomy and prior hysterectomy worst QoL -Loose or watery stool was not a factor for increased MMHQ scores

Table 1.
What do we know about QoL in patients with FI?

Some years after the development of the FIQL scale, Bordeianou and Rockwood published a prospective analysis of the correlation between severity and QoL, using two tools designed for the same group, the FISI for severity and the FIQL scale, and also the SF-36 [42]. All the domains of the FIQL were significantly altered, being coping-behaviour and embarrassment the two most affected sub-scales. Furthermore, SF-36 scores decreased as the severity of FI increased, with the exception of the scales on pain, physical role and physical functioning, which was expectable as usually alterations in the QoL of patients with FI are social and emotional. Moreover, the authors reviewed the SF-36 alterations in other chronic diseases managed in an outpatient setting and reported that patients with FI were worse than those with rheumatoid arthritis or diabetes, and as severely affected as patients with inflammatory bowel disease.

Since the publication of the FIQL scale, most studies have used this tool to measure the QoL in FI. Bharucha et al. [31] mailed a questionnaire to an age-stratified random sample of 5300 women treated at two primary care centres covering 80% of a population of 100.000 inhabitants. Subjects with FI during the previous year were assessed by a symptom severity validated scale (Fecal Incontinence and Constipation Assessment, FICA) [30] and a QoL scale consisting in 15 domains adapted from the FIQL scale. The survey was answered by 2800 women and the prevalence of FI was 18.5%. FI had a moderate or severe impact on one or more of the 15 QoL domains in 23% of the women with FI. The study demonstrated that urgency affects more QoL than passive FI alone, being worse if both types of FI are associated, probably due to the anxiety generated by the urgency. Interestingly, women with less than one episode of leakage per month had more impact on their QoL than those patients with the lowest QoL. Furthermore, they found that scores for activities in which toilet access was unpredictable (i.e. going to the cinema, shopping, recreational activities or sports, leaving home, travelling by car, plane or train) and for activities that involved eating (i.e. eating before leaving home, going out to eat) were higher (indicating worse QoL) than scores for activities associated with predictable toilet access (i.e. employment, working home, sex life, visiting friends or relatives, staying overnight away from home and family relationships).

Boreham [43] studied FI in 457 women presenting for gynaecologic care on benign conditions, and reported that prevalence of FI was 28.4%. Moreover, even when the authors considered FI that had an impact on the QoL (answering anything except "never" on the FIQL scale), the prevalence of FI reached 21.7%. Of the 130 women with FI, 76.2% scored very low in the FIQL scales, being also embarrassment the most affected domain. Women with liquid stool leakages reported the largest impact on QoL. Another important aspect that impacts the QoL of patients with FI is the feeling that they are compelled to adapt to their poor situation for the rest of their lives. This study showed several interesting facts: (a) almost three quarters of women reported that FI symptoms were present for 3 years or less; (b) only 11.4% of them had previously sought care; (c) predictors of health care seeking included loss of solid stool and lower scores on the FIQL embarrassment scale and (d) 44.7% of women thought that there was no treatment available.

The findings of this study explain why this condition has been referred to as "the silent affliction" or "the unvoiced symptom" [46, 47] because of the associated stigma. Moreover, we must consider that the overall prevalence of FI is also underestimated because health professionals do not ask about this problem. Aitola et al. reported that only 27% of patients had discussed FI with their physician [48]. Dunivan et al. found that 36% of primary care patients reported FI but only 2.7% carried FI as a medical diagnosis, thus suggesting a lack of knowledge by health professionals [49].

Bartlett and colleagues [50] studied the major reasons for non-disclosure of FI symptoms in patients attending a urogynaecology and colorectal clinic for other conditions. They identified that main reasons were: FI historical but not current; problem not considered as FI by the patient; administrated questionnaires too long; embarrassing condition; doctor considered too busy; patient wanted to focus on the primary reason for consultation and the doctor explained that a one-off bout of uncontrollable diarrhoea was not FI. Nevertheless, interviewees reported that patients would respond to FI questions initiated by their general practitioner during regular consultations.

Later on, the same group [44] reported that more than 22% of patients that attended urogynaecology and colorectal clinic for other conditions than FI, had a QoL severely affected by FI in all four scales. Factors affecting the QoL were increased bowel frequency, quantity of fecal loss, type of incontinence and fecal urgency. Patients with both solid and liquid incontinence reported a poorer QoL than those with either only solid or liquid incontinent episodes. Given the relationship between the FIQL scales and the quantity of fecal leakage, the authors suggested that the quantity of fecal loss as well as frequency, type, urgency and pad wearing should be included in the definition of FI severity [44]. Another interesting aspect of this study was the small difference found in the FIQL scales when comparing weekly and monthly incontinence episodes, as other authors have previously reported [29], probably because infrequent incontinence episode are always unexpected, and hence, similarly distressing.

Several studies have assessed a potential difference between genders concerning the impact on QoL, with women experiencing a greater impact when compared with men [51, 52]. However, this has not been supported by other reports which failed to find significant differences [44, 53].

Studies using other scales such as MMHQ have been also reached interesting conclusions. Markland [45] studied women presenting with FI and reported a weak correlation between the FISI severity score and the MMHQ. Younger women (<65 years) had higher MMHQ scores, representing a negative impact on HRQoL and the authors suggested that young patients were more likely to report their limitations and seek treatment. However, other studies found that older women had worse QoL than younger women, and justified that a delay in treatment resulted in poorer QoL [50]. Thus, further studies are needed to address the impact on QOL depending on the age. In the same study [45], increased bowel movements and urgency were associated with significantly higher MMHQ scores. After controlling for age and comorbid disease, women reporting more bowel urgency had increased MMHQ score. Urinary incontinence, prior cholecystectomy and prior hysterectomy were also associated with increased QoL scores. Interestingly, loose stool or diarrhea was not a significant factor for increased MMHQ scores in the multivariate analysis.

A prospective study including women with FI investigated the relationship with depression and abdominal pain [54]. Depression was assessed by the Patient Health Questionnaire (PHQ) [55]. Diabetes, prior hysterectomy, abdominal pain, history of previous health care for FI and higher FISI scores were associated with more severe QoL scores. Furthermore, higher PHQ scores predicted worse QoL scores overall and in all four of the FIQL subscales. Other studies have reported a relation between FI and depression [56]. This is an important fact to take into account, because patients with FI are required to cooperate in the management plan, and those suffering from major depression will be less likely to follow a rigorous program. Obviously, FI itself may be the main factor for a depression status; therefore, being aware of it and helping patients is likely to improve the overall treatment.

A study [57] with a cross-sectional design including 2269 ethnically diverse women aged 40–80 years, investigated the impact of FI on sexual QoL. The majority (60%) was sexually active despite having FI, but their sexual function was impaired. The multivariate analysis showed that women with FI experienced significantly lower sexual desire, lower sexual satisfaction, and limitation of sexual activity. Women with isolated gas incontinence reported sexual functioning similar to women without FI. The authors concluded that sexual life should be evaluated and prioritized during therapeutic management, as it is important to women with FI.

In conclusion, key points could be summarized as follows:

1. FI is a frequent condition with a higher prevalence of that reported in previous studies.

2. FI has been a neglected problem worldwide. Reasons for non-disclosure and non-detected FI are multifactorial and related to the fear of embarrassment, but also to the lack of professionals dealing with the problem.

3. QoL of patients with FI is severely affected in almost all life domains.

4. The FIQL scale seems to be a useful and essential tool to assess QoL. Alterations in almost all domains have been demonstrated, especially in coping and embarrassment scales.

5. The relationship between severity and QoL in FI is a complex matter, but it has been suggested that the quantity of loss, bowel urgency and increased bowel frequency should be measured and taken into account.

6. More specific aspects, such as depression or sexual activity, should also be introduced in the evaluation of these patients in order to improve the quality of health care.

6. Is the improvement of patients treated for FI reflected enough in the QOL scales?

For the last 10 years, most studies regarding FI treatments have analyzed its impact on QOL. The FIQL scale has been the most used score to evidence such improvement, thus responsiveness of this score has been widely demonstrated.

A systematic review [58] about outcomes after anal sphincter repair showed that, although continence deteriorates in the long-term, QoL and satisfaction remained relatively high. The scales used in the studies were heterogeneous and, despite most studies were published after the development of the specific QoL scores, less than half used them.

Since the first multicentre European study about the feasibility of sacral neuromodulation [59], most centres regularly use the FIQL scale and some of them also add the SF-36. Consequently, most articles on this treatment mention the improvement in the four domains of the FIQL scale correlating with the FI improvement, as well as some changes in the generic questionnaire. However, few studies go deeper into the details of the meaning of these changes.

A report about the long-term outcome and QoL in patients treated by sacral neuromodulation showed a significant and stable improvement in all four categories of the FIQL scale, in contrast to the SF-36 score, which only showed a significant improvement in the social functioning, emotional and mental health subscales, probably due to its generic profile [60]. On the other hand, other studies have demonstrated the quick onset on this QoL improvement, which is already present at 3 months follow-up [61–63].

The Sacral Nerve Stimulation Study Group in the USA [64] reported in-depth details about changes in QoL from baseline through 4 years of follow-up. They reported that not only the four FIQL scales were significantly improved but there was also an improvement in each of the component questions. Before the treatment, patients tended to stay close to a toilet, thought about the impact of food on their bowel function, disliked their body image, and were very limited in their personal intimate life. After sacral neuromodulation, less patients were worried about the proximity to a toilet, were fearful to sleep elsewhere than at home, avoided travelling by plane or train, disliked their body image. Patients also reported an improvement in their sexual life. Moreover, patient-reported overall health was significantly improved, demonstrating a general perception of improvement in wellbeing beyond the mere restoration of continence. Furthermore, they demonstrated that Embarrassment and Copying-Behaviour were the most affected dimensions, and that correlated better with clinical improvement than Depression and Lifestyle subscales. This fact could be explained because even if patients are not fully continent, their QoL is better secondary to less episodes of FI, but they still remain affected by all the changes that altered their lives during the time that they suffered FI.

Other reports have highlighted the impact of different surgical treatments, such as injectable bulking agents, artificial bowel sphincter or dynamic graciloplasty, on the QOL of patients with FI [44].

7. Measuring patient satisfaction

The current role of clinicians has changed from helping patients through their illness, to have higher expectations that include both cure and alleviate chronic symptoms. Moreover, patients tend to be active consumers of health care, so they may participate on the medical decision-making. On the other hand, monitoring treatment results is mandatory in current practice. For all these reasons, the QoL scales should be used, at least when treatment outcomes are measured.

Nevertheless, the question is whether they are practical and whether its use in the clinical practice is realistic. On certain occasions, decisions based on clinical improvement and patient satisfaction need to be made, and sometimes is impossible to score a QOL scale, in the outpatients' clinic context.

Some studies have reported simple ways to measure patient satisfaction, which are complementary to the application of QOL scores. This implies the addition of study-specific customized questions, typically focusing on subjective measures of satisfaction or QOL (i.e. "Would you recommend a sphincteroplasty to a friend?" or "Are you pleased with the results of your surgery?"). Other authors have used a Likert Scale or Visual Analogue Scales (VAS) to measure patient's satisfaction with the outcome [58].

A study [28] measuring the efficacy of different tools used in FI patient's evaluation, demonstrated and excellent intra and interobserver reliability of both CCCS and St Mark's score. Moreover, all domains of the FIQL demonstrate excellent intraobserver reliability, although a simple quality of life assessment tool such as VAS still maintains a better intraobserver agreement.

The relationship between patient's satisfaction and clinical outcome, assessed by bowel diaries and symptom scores, was evaluated in a study on sacral neuromodulation [65]. Patients were asked to indicate if they were satisfied with their current treatment results, with a simple question (yes/no) that simplified the analysis of predictive factors of outcome. It was evident that this relationship is complex and does not match the traditional used success criteria.

In another study [64], patients were asked to rate his/her own bowel health on a scale from 0 to 10, 0 indicating the worst imaginable situation and a 10 indicating the best one.

There is no consensus on what is the best way to measure patient satisfaction easily, but it is clear that the way to evaluate patients must improve and its validation must be a future line of research.

8. Final comments

Traditionally, it has been assumed that testing is essential in the evaluation of FI. Anorectal manometry and anal ultrasound have been considered the most useful and available tests to assess FI. Investigations would be clearly useful for patients with a sphincter injury that could benefit from surgical repair. However, in daily practice, the reality for the majority of patients is that testing rarely helps in the decision-making, as decisions are mainly based on the patient's symptoms. It is commonly known that some patients with mild clinical symptoms may have a severe dysfunction when tested, and on the contrary, there are patients experiencing severe FI but showing minor structural and functional alterations. Moreover, treatment decisions and outcome evaluation after treatment should not be decided only considering the symptom severity but the impact on QOL and the patient satisfaction. Finally, considering the economic cost of some of the current treatments for FI, changes in QoL should be demonstrated before implementing certain procedures.

Society is evolving, which implies changes in lifestyle and the possibility of new treatments in the future. Therefore, it might be necessary to rethink the way of assessing QoL, and that questionnaires will need to evolve as well, to adapt to the new circumstances. Readers must be encouraged to become familiar with QoL instruments and their limitations.

Acknowledgements

Laura Lagares-Tena has contributed extensively in the edition of this chapter. No funds have been used to this chapter.

Conflict of interest

The authors declare no conflicts of interest.

Nomenclature

FI	fecal incontinence
QoL	quality of life
HRQoL	health-related quality of life
IQOLA	international quality of life assessment
SF-36	short form 36 health status questionnaire
FIQL	fecal incontinence quality of life scale
GIQLI	gastrointestinal quality of life index
MHQ	Manchester health questionnaire
MMHQ	modified Manchester health questionnaire
FISI	fecal incontinence severity scale
CCCS	Cleveland Clinic continence score
FICA	fecal incontinence and constipation assessment
ICIQ-B	international consultation on incontinence questionnaire–bowel symptoms
DQO	direct questionning of objectives
PHQ	patient health questionnaire
VAS	visual analogue scales

Author details

Arantxa Muñoz Duyos[1*] and Yolanda Ribas[2]

1 University Hospital Mútua Terrassa, Barcelona University, Terrassa, Barcelona, Spain

2 Consorci Sanitari de Terrassa, Terrassa, Spain

*Address all correspondence to: amduyos@gmail.com

IntechOpen

References

[1] The WHOQOL Group. Development of the World Health Organization WHOQOL-BREF quality of life assessment. Psychological Medicine. 1998;**28**(3):551-558

[2] Testa MA, Simonson DC. Assesment of quality-of-life outcomes. The New England Journal of Medicine. 1996;**334**(13):835-840

[3] U.S Department of Health and Human Services Food and Drug Administration Guidance for Industry: Patient-Reported Outcome Measures: Use in Medical Product Development to Support Labeling Claims. U.S. FDA, Clinical/Medical. 2009. Available form: http://www.fda.gov/downloads/Drugs/GuidanceComplianceRegulatoryInformation/Guidances/UCM193282.pdf

[4] Acquadro C, Berzon R, Dubois D, Leidy NK, Marquis P, Revicki D, et al. Incorporating the patient's perspective into drug development and communication: an ad hoc task force report of the patient-reported outcomes (PRO) Harmonization Group meeting at the Food and Drug Administration, February 16, 2001. Value in Health. 2003;**6**(5):522-531

[5] Faecal incontinence in adults: management. NICE Clinical guideline [CG49] Publisheddate. 2007. Available from: https://www.nice.org.uk/guidance/cg49/chapter/1-Guidance

[6] Whitehead WE. Diagnosing and managing fecal incontinence: if you don"t ask, they won"t tell. Gastroenterology. 2005;**129**(1):6

[7] Christensen AI, Ekholm O, Glümer C, Juel K. Effect of survey mode on response patterns: comparison of face-to-face and self-administered modes in health surveys. European Journal of Public Health. 2014;**24**(2):327-332

[8] Bandayrel K, Johnston BC. Recent advances in patient and proxy-reported quality of life research. Health and Quality of Life Outcomes. 2014;**12**:110

[9] Hwang HF, Chen CY, Lin MR. Patient-proxy agreement on the health-related quality of life one year after traumatic brain injury. Archives of Physical Medicine and Rehabilitation. 2017;**98**(12):2540-2547

[10] Eiser C, Varni JW. Health-related quality of life and symptom reporting: similarities and differences between children and their parents. European Journal of Pediatrics. 2013;**172**(10):1299-1304

[11] Ravens-Sieberer U, Erhart M, Rajmil L, Herdman M, Auquier P, Bruil J, et al. European KIDSCREEN Group. Reliability, construct and criterion validity of the KIDSCREEN-10 score: a short measure for children and adolescents' well-being and health-related quality of life. Quality of Life Research. 2010;**19**(10):1487-1500

[12] American Educational Research Association. American Psychological Association, National Council on Measurement in Education. Standards for Educational and Psychological Testing. Washington, DC: American Educational Research Association; 1999

[13] Bullinger M, Alonso J, Apolone G, Leplège A, Sullivan M, Wood-Dauphinee S, et al. Translating health status questionnaires and evaluating their quality: the IQOLA Project approach. International Quality of Life Assessment. Journal of Clinical Epidemiology. 1998;**51**(11):913-923

[14] Sperber AD. Translation and validation of study instruments for cross-cultural research. Gastroenterology. 2004;**126**(Suppl 1): S124-S128

[15] Ware JE, Sherbourne CD. The MOS 36-item short-form health survey (SF-36). I. Conceptual framework and item selection. Medical Care. 1992;**30**(6):473-483

[16] Elsenbruch S, Harnish MJ, Orr WC. Subjective and objective sleep quality in irritable bowel syndrome. The American Journal of Gastroenterology. 1999;**94**(9):2447-2452

[17] Vrijens D, Berghmans B, Nieman F, van Os J, van Koeveringe G, Leue C. Prevalence of anxiety and depressive symptoms and their association with pelvic floor dysfunctions–A cross sectional cohort study at a Pelvic Care Centre. Neurourology and Urodynamics. 2017;**36**(7):1816-1823

[18] Rockwood TH. Incontinence severity and QOL scales for fecal incontinence. Gastroenterology. 2004;**126**(Suppl 1):S106-S113

[19] Rockwood TH, Church JM, Fleshman JW, Kane RL, Mavrantonis C, Thorson AG, et al. Fecal incontinence quality of life scale: Quality of life instrument for patients with fecal incontinence. Diseases of the Colon & Rectum. 2000;**43**(1):9-16; discussion 16-7

[20] Eypasch E, Williams JI, Wood-Dauphinee S, Ure BM, Schmülling C, Neugebauer E, et al. Gastrointestinal quality of life index: development, validation and application of a new instrument. The British Journal of Surgery. 1995;**82**(2):216-222

[21] Bugg G, Kiff E, Hosker G. A new condition-specific health-related quality of life questionnaire for the assessment of women with anal incontinence. British Journal of Obstetrics and Gynaecology;**108**:1057-1067

[22] Kelleher CJ, Cardozo LD, Khullar V, Salvatore S. A new questionnaire to assess the quality of life of urinary incontinent women. British Journal of Obstetrics and Gynaecology. 1997;**104**(12):1374-1379

[23] Kwon S, Visco AG, Fitzgerald MP, Ye W, Whitehead WE. Validity and reliability of the modified manchester health questionnaire in assessing patients with fecal incontinence. Diseases of the Colon and Rectum. 2005;**48**(2):323-334

[24] Pescatori M, Anastasio G, Bottini C, Mentasti A. New grading and scoring for anal incontinence. Evaluation of 335 patients. Diseases of the Colon & Rectum. 1992;**35**(5):482-487

[25] Parks AG. Royal society of medicine, section of proctology; meeting 27 November 1974. President's address. Anorectal incontinence. Proceedings of the Royal Society of Medicine. 1975;**68**(11):681-690

[26] Jorge JM, Wexner SD. Etiology and management of fecal incontinence. Diseases of the Colon and Rectum. 1993;**36**(1):77-97

[27] Vaizey CJ, Carapeti E, Cahill JA, Kamm MA. Prospective comparison of faecal incontinence grading systems. Gut. 1999;**44**(1):77-80

[28] Hussain ZI, Lim M, Stojkovic S. The test-retest reliability of fecal incontinence severity and quality-of-life assessment tools. Diseases of the Colon and Rectum. 2014;**57**(5):638-644

[29] Rockwood TH, Church JM, Fleshman JW, Kane RL, Mavrantonis C, Thorson AG, et al. Patient and surgeon ranking of the severity of symptoms associated with fecal incontinence: the fecal incontinence severity index. Diseases of the Colon and Rectum. 1999;**42**(12):1525-1532

[30] Bharucha AE, Locke GR, Seide BM, Zinsmeister AR. A new questionnaire for constipation and faecal

incontinence. Alimentary Pharmacology & Therapeutics. 2004;**20**(3):355-364

[31] Bharucha AE, Zinsmeister AR, Locke GR, Schleck C, McKeon K, Melton LJ. Symptoms and quality of life in community women with fecal incontinence. Clinical Gastroenterology and Hepatology. 2006;**4**(8):1004-1009

[32] Baxter NN, Rothenberger DA, Lowry AC. Measuring fecal incontinence. Diseases of the Colon and Rectum. 2003;**46**(12):1591-1605

[33] Rockwood T. Are you worried about bowel accidents? Quality of life in fecal incontinence. Diseases of the Colon and Rectum. 2008;**51**(9):1434

[34] Peterson AC, Sutherland JM, Liu G, Crump RT, Karimuddin AA. Evaluation of the fecal incontinence quality of life scale (FIQL) using item response theory reveals limitations and suggests revisions. Quality of Life Research. 2018;**27**(6):1613-1623

[35] Cotterill N, Norton C, Avery KNL, Abrams P, Donovan JL. A patient-centered approach to developing a comprehensive symptom and quality of life assessment of anal incontinence. Diseases of the Colon and Rectum. 2008;**51**(1):82-87

[36] Wexner SD, Baeten C, Bailey R, Bakka A, Belin B, Belliveau P, et al. Long-term efficacy of dynamic graciloplasty for fecal incontinence. Diseases of the Colon and Rectum. 2002;**45**(6):809-818

[37] Byrne CM, Pager CK, Rex J, Roberts R, Solomon MJ. Assessment of quality of life in the treatment of patients with neuropathic fecal incontinence. Diseases of the Colon and Rectum. 2002;**45**(11):1431-1436

[38] Lee JT, Madoff RD, Rockwood TH. Quality-of-life measures in fecal incontinence: is validation valid? Diseases of the Colon and Rectum. 2015;**58**:352-357

[39] O'Keefe EA, Talley NJ, Zinsmeister AR, Jacobsen SJ. Bowel disorders impair functional status and quality of life in the elderly: A population-based study. The Journals of Gerontology Series A: Biological Sciences and Medical Sciences. 1995;**50A**(4):M184-M189

[40] Edwards NI, Jones D. The prevalence of faecal incontinence in older people living at home. Age and Ageing. 2001;**30**(6):503-507

[41] Perry S, Shaw C, McGrother C, Matthews RJ, Assassa RP, Dallosso H, et al. Prevalence of faecal incontinence in adults aged 40 years or more living in the community. Gut. 2002;**50**(4):480-484

[42] Bordeianou L, Rockwood T, Baxter N, Lowry A, Mellgren A, Parker S. Does incontinence severity correlate with quality of life? Prospective analysis of 502 consecutive patients. Colorectal Disease. 2008;**10**(3):273-279

[43] Boreham MK, Richter HE, Kenton KS, Nager CW, Gregory WT, Aronson MP, et al. Anal incontinence in women presenting for gynecologic care: Prevalence, risk factors, and impact upon quality of life. American Journal of Obstetrics and Gynecology. 2005;**192**(5):1637-1642

[44] Bartlett L. Impact of fecal incontinence on quality of life. World Journal of Gastroenterology. 2009;**15**(26):3276-3282

[45] Markland AD, Greer WJ, Vogt A, Redden DT, Goode PS, Burgio KL, et al. Factors impacting quality of life in women with fecal incontinence. Diseases of the Colon and Rectum. 2010;**53**(8):1148-1154

[46] Johanson JF, Lafferty J. Epidemiology of fecal incontinence: the silent affliction. The American Journal of Gastroenterology. 1996;**91**(1):33-36

[47] Leigh RJ, Turnberg LA. Faecal incontinence: the unvoiced symptom. Lancet. 1982;**1**(8285):1349-1351

[48] Aitola P, Lehto K, Fonsell R, Huhtala H. Prevalence of faecal incontinence in adults aged 30 years or more in general population. Colorect Disease. 2010;**12**(7):687-691

[49] Dunivan GC, Heymen S, Palsson OS, Korff M, Turner MJ, Melville JL, et al. Fecal incontinence in primary care: prevalence, diagnosis, and health care utilization. American Journal of Obstetrics and Gynecology. 2010;**202**(5):493.e1-493.e6

[50] Bartlett L, Nowak M, Ho YH. Reasons for non-disclosure of faecal incontinence: a comparison between two survey methods. Techniques in Coloproctology. 2007;**11**(3):251-257

[51] Alsheik EH, Coyne T, Hawes SK, et al. Fecal incontinence: prevalence, severity, and quality of life data from an outpatient gastroenterology practice. Gastroenterology Research and Practice. 2012;**2012**:947694

[52] Cohan JN, Chou AB, Varma MG. Fecal incontinence in men referred for specialty care: a cross-sectional study. Colorectal Disease. 2015;**17**:802-809

[53] Christoforidis D, Bordeianou L, Rockwood TH, Lowry AC, Parker S, Mellgren AF. Fecal incontinence in men. Colorectal Disease. 2011;**13**:906-913

[54] Smith TM, Menees SB, Xu X, Saad RJ, Chey WD, Fenner DE. Factors associated with quality of life among women with fecal incontinence. International Urogynecology Journal. 2012;**24**(3):493-499

[55] Kroenke K, Spitzer RL, Williams JB. The PHQ-9: validity of a brief depression severity measure. Journal of General Internal Medicine. 2001;**16**(9):606-613

[56] Crowell MD, Schettler VA, Lacy BE, Lunsford TN, Harris LA, DiBaise JK, et al. Impact of anal incontinence on psychosocial function and health-related quality of life. Digestive Diseases and Sciences. 2007;**52**(7):1627-1631

[57] Imhoff LR, Brown JS, Creasman JM, Subak LL, Van Den Eeden SK, Thom DH, et al. Fecal incontinence decreases sexual quality of life, but does not prevent sexual activity in women. Diseases of the Colon and Rectum. 2012;**55**(10):1059-1065

[58] Glasgow SC, Lowry AC. Long-term outcomes of anal sphincter repair for fecal incontinence: a systematic review. Diseases of the Colon and Rectum. 2012;**55**(4):482-490

[59] Matzel KE, Kamm MA, Stösser M, Baeten CGMI, Christiansen J, Madoff R, et al. Sacral spinal nerve stimulation for faecal incontinence: multicentre study. Lancet. 2004;**363**(9417):1270-1276

[60] Uludağ O, Melenhorst J, Koch SM, Gemert WG, Dejong CHC, Baeten CG. Sacral neuromodulation: Long-term outcome and quality of life in patients with faecal incontinence. Colorect Disease. 2011;**13**(10):1162-1166

[61] Ripetti V, Caputo D, Ausania F, Esposito E, Bruni R, Arullani A. Sacral nerve neuromodulation improves physical, psychological and social quality of life in patients with fecal incontinence. Techniques in Coloproctology. 2002;**6**(3):147-152

[62] Uludağ O, Koch SMP, van Gemert WG, Dejong CHC, Baeten CGMI. Sacral neuromodulation: Long-term outcome and quality of life in patients with faecal

incontinence. Colorectal Disease. 2011;**13**(10):1162-1166

[63] Leroi A-M, Parc Y, Lehur P-A, Mion F, Barth X, Rullier E, et al. Efficacy of sacral nerve stimulation for fecal incontinence: results of a multicenter double-blind crossover study. Annals of Surgery. 2005;**242**(5):662-669

[64] Devroede G, Giese C, Wexner SD, Mellgren A, Coller JA, Madoff RD, et al. Quality of life is markedly improved in patients with fecal incontinence after sacral nerve stimulation. Female Pelvic Medicine & Reconstructive Surgery. 2012;**18**(2):103-112

[65] Duelund-Jakobsen J, van Wunnik B, Buntzen S, Lundby L, Laurberg S, Baeten C. Baseline factors predictive of patient satisfaction with sacral neuromodulation for idiopathic fecal incontinence. International Journal of Colorectal Disease. 2014;**29**(7):793-798

Section 3

Faecal Incontinence and Disorders of Evacuation

Chapter 4

Assessment and Treatment of Obstructed Defecation Syndrome

Dimitrios Linardoutsos

Abstract

Fecal incontinence is not a rare clinical pathology in general population. Although it is more common in geriatric population, fecal incontinence should not be underestimated in younger genders. Obstructive defecation syndrome (ODS) has become a well-known syndrome with different clinical etiology and symptoms. The main symptom is inability of proper rectal emptying, but it can also overlap with symptoms of incontinence. In this chapter, we emphasize on the assessment of ODS, focusing on the coexistence and clinical relation to fecal incontinence. Anorectal studies are of great importance for the evaluation of the symptoms. Biofeedback is the key to the proper management of patients with ODS, showing significant improvement in incontinence as well. Surgical treatment of anatomic deformities that cause ODS is also important.

Keywords: obstructive defecation syndrome, incontinence, rectocele, dyssynergia, biofeedback

1. Introduction

Fecal incontinence is a common clinical problem in general population, mainly in older people. By definition, it is the inability to control bowel movements or, in other words, the uncontrolled and involuntary loss of solid or liquid stool or gas. The uncontrolled loss should last at least more than 1 month and with regard to patients who were previously continent. The terms anal or bowel incontinence are also used to represent the same clinical entity. Fecal incontinence, as a symptom, has various etiologies. Obstructed defecation syndrome is a very common pathology acting actually as one of the underlying causes of fecal incontinence.

Obstructed defecation syndrome (ODS) is the inability of the patient to empty the rectum normally. By definition, it is a clinical condition where the patient has the feeling of not emptying the rectum adequately. It can also be related, sometimes, to reduced bowel movements. Terminology of this condition in the literature also includes rectal outlet obstruction or evacuatory dysfunction. ODS may coexist with other bowel pathologies such as irritable bowel syndrome, anatomical deformities such as sigmoidocele, or even other colonic motility disorders, such as slow transit constipation. ODS is frequently associated with fecal incontinence. The established status quo is that fecal impaction, as a secondary effect from a rectocele or intussusception, causes overflow incontinence. Prolonged fecal impaction, prolapse or other ODS pathologies, all contribute to impairment of rectal compliance and thus sensitivity, as well as sphincter damage from chronic distention. ODS from various causes can provoke episodes of incontinence; however, new data suggest an increased risk of anal incontinence in patients who have had different types of operation for ODS in the past.

2. Defecation physiology

In order to understand the physiology of defecation, deep knowledge of the anatomy of the rectum and anal canal is very important. The rectum is the last part of the large intestine, located in the lower pelvis. Rectal function is crucial for retention of stool (continence) and for evacuation (defecation). The rectum measures about 15–17 cm in length, descending along the sacrococcygeal concavity and passing through the pelvic floor to the anal canal. The major part is called the rectal ampulla, which is a wide segment, with a perimeter that can extend to more than 15 cm. The lowest and narrowest part is the anal canal. The anorectal junction is formatted by the constant traction of the puborectal sling. The levator ani muscle, formed by the iliococcygeus, the pubococcygeal, and the puborectal muscles, serves as the pelvic floor. The relaxation of levator ani, and mainly the puborectalis muscle, the perineum and contraction of the lower abdomen, and the relaxation of the anal sphincter, all work in tandem in order to provide a normal defecation. Distention of rectal wall stimulates contractions of colon and rectal wall, mediated by the parasympathetic defecation reflex. Thus, phasic rectal contractions start and tone increases, formatting a conduit shape of rectum rather than a reservoir. For the above pattern of function, rectal sensitivity is of great importance. Once the rectum is filled with stool, the internal anal sphincter relaxes, as per the rectoanal inhibitory reflex. Simultaneous relaxation of the puborectalis muscle creates an obtuse anorectal angle, thus allowing defecation to occur normally. Defecation can be postponed with voluntary contraction of the external anal sphincter. Regarding pelvic floor innervations, the pudendal nerve innervates the external anal sphincter and some fibers of the puborectalis muscle, while the rest of puborectalis and levator ani muscles are getting innervations from sacral roots of S3 and S4 [1].

3. Clinical manifestation

Symptoms of ODS include rectal or lower abdominal pain, a feeling of bloatedness or incomplete rectal evacuation, the use of vaginal splitting or perineal manipulation to help the defecation, prolonged straining, spending more time than usual in toilet, perineal descent, report of hard stools as well as dependency on laxatives and enemas. Obstructive defecation syndrome may be of various functional or anatomical origins. Functional etiology includes aganglionic rectum (short-term Hirschsprung), neuropathic disorders (multiple sclerosis, spinal cord lesions), and pelvic floor dyssynergia, such as in anismic patients. Mechanical ODS comes from anatomic deformities such as internal intussusception, rectocele, rectal prolapse or enterocele [2].

Soiling and real fecal incontinence are also usual symptoms of ODS mainly, but not solely, representing overflow diarrhea. In this chapter, we will focus on the coexistence and clinical relation between obstructive defecation syndrome and fecal incontinence.

4. Epidemiology

Obstructive defecation and fecal incontinence have been recognized as related pathologies in geriatric population [3]. Fecal impaction and concomitant overflow diarrhea, as a typical non-controlled loss of stool, is not unusual. However, the coexistence of other pathologies and the lack of accurate statistics still exist [4]. Fecal impaction and chronic straining can cause denervation and pelvic floor weakness, which is the most well-known cause of obstructed defecation syndrome [5].

Apart from chronic straining as a known cause, adaptation of endoanal ultrasound in assessment of incontinence showed anal sphincter disruption as a common cause of fecal incontinence [6]. However, it is well known that prevalence of anal incontinence remains equal between genders. This leads to the possible conclusion that the role of obstetric injury in fecal incontinence is important, but may be not crucial, bearing in mind the equal number of male patients suffering from this condition. In addition, most female patients who suffer from incontinence, report the onset of their symptoms many years after delivery, making clinicians consider other contributing pathologies on top of the sphincter damage [7]. Recently, more studies are dealing with the coexistence of underlying constipation and fecal pathology [8].

In general, population, overlapping of symptoms of slow transit constipation, obstructive defecation, and incontinence are considerable, indicating constipation as a principal risk factor for fecal incontinence. Damon et al. found that between 706 patients, 63% reported difficulty in defecation, and 51% found to have sense of incomplete evacuation [9]. Several other studies represent similar findings and demonstrate the role of ODS in coexistent fecal incontinence [10, 11].

More specifically, in patients assessed in colorectal clinics, although the series are small, proctographic studies have shown similar findings. Rex et al. used anorectal manometry and defecography for the assessment of their patients. They demonstrated retention of contrast in rectoceles and incomplete evacuation in patients having clinical symptoms of ODS with concurrent incontinence [12]. In another study by Harewood et al., between 38 patients that evaluated with symptoms of incomplete evacuation and straining, 15% were found to also suffer from fecal incontinence [13]. In another study from Mohammed SD et al. on 200 patients complaining for symptoms of ODS, 91% reported incontinence [14]. Similar reports are coming from an evaluation of 161 male patients complaining for fecal incontinence, having found that almost half of them (48%) have concurrent functional constipation [15].

5. Assessment

Rectal function and defecation should be assessed clinically and with several radiological or functional tests. Apart from colonoscopy, which is important to exclude any malignant causes of changes in bowel habits, clinical examination may reveal descent perineum, absence of rectoanal inhibitor reflex, sphincter tears or external openings of perianal sinus. Observation of perineum after requesting patient to squeeze usually allows us to understand if intussusception, or prolapse, is the clinical problem. Digital rectal exam is crucial to estimate the rest and squeeze anal tone, to assess for possible fecal impaction, rectocele or to palpate any abnormal mass.

Rectal sensitivity is usually assessed with air or water insufflation and distention of either a balloon or condom inserted to the rectum. Today multimodal balloon catheters allow the analysis of electrical and temperature receptors as well. Balloon expansion resembles the full rectum and triggers the need for evacuation. The time, the volume of the balloon, and the difficulty to expel provide much information about the rectal sensitivity and the possible dyssynergic defecation. Mean balloon volume is 50 ml of water. Expulsion should take less than 30 s in young men and less than 1 min in older men, but in women expulsion should occur in about a minute, regardless of age. Balloon expulsion test along with anorectal manometry is considered the primary diagnostic tests for identifying ODS. New manometric catheters have an expulsion balloon on the tip, permitting the performance of anorectal manometry at the same time. Anorectal manometry with high resolution catheters provides excellent information. Catheters can have up to 36 channels, evaluating pressure along the entire anal canal as long as the changes of pressures at the time of rectal distention (**Figure 1**). Physicians can get information for rest and squeeze pressures, about the rectoanal inhibitor reflex, the push defecation test, and the pressures during cough.

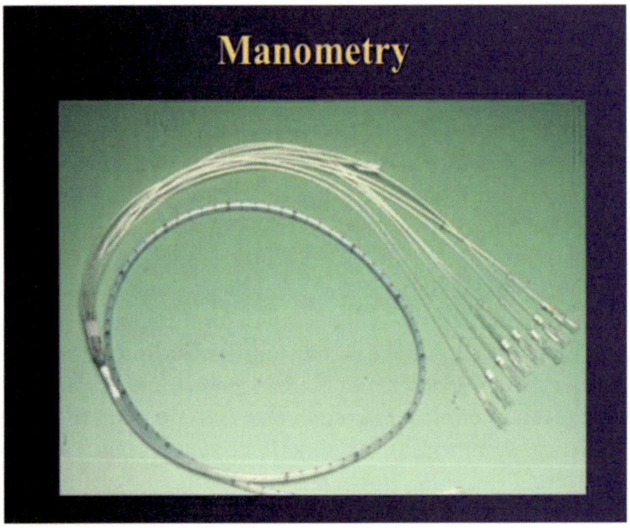

Figure 1.
Anorectal manometry catheter. The multiple respective channels can be seen.

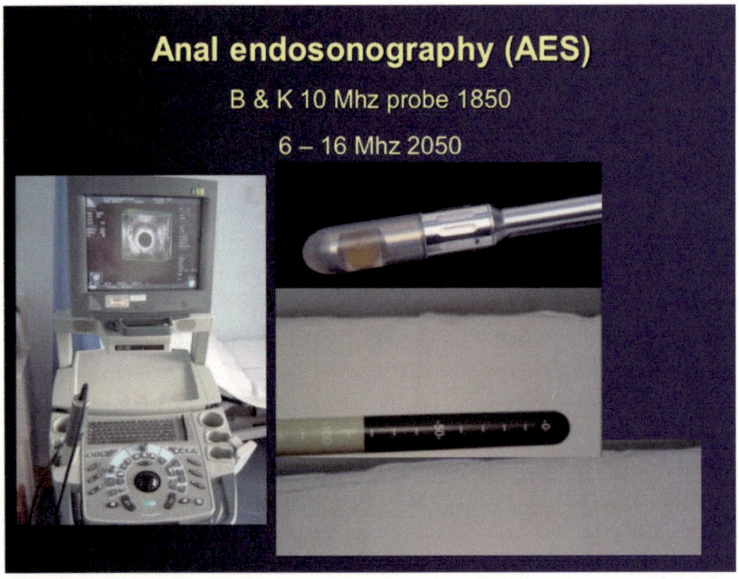

Figure 2.
Anal endosonography equipment. The ultrasound can be seen in operation at the left, while the ultrasound probe can be seen on the right.

Anorectal ultrasonography is the most useful test not only to estimate the anatomy of the anal sphincters but also to estimate possible enterocele or rectocele, using the proper probe for perineal view (**Figures 2–4**). It is a cheap, painless, and very informative exam and provides the information needed by a colorectal surgeon. In expert hands, it can be the only exam necessary to evaluate obstructive defecation syndrome. Although most of the information taken from a proctogram can also be deciphered from a good total anorectal and pelvic ultrasound, experts in most centers prefer a combination of both for the best assessment of the patient [16] (**Figures 5** and **6**).

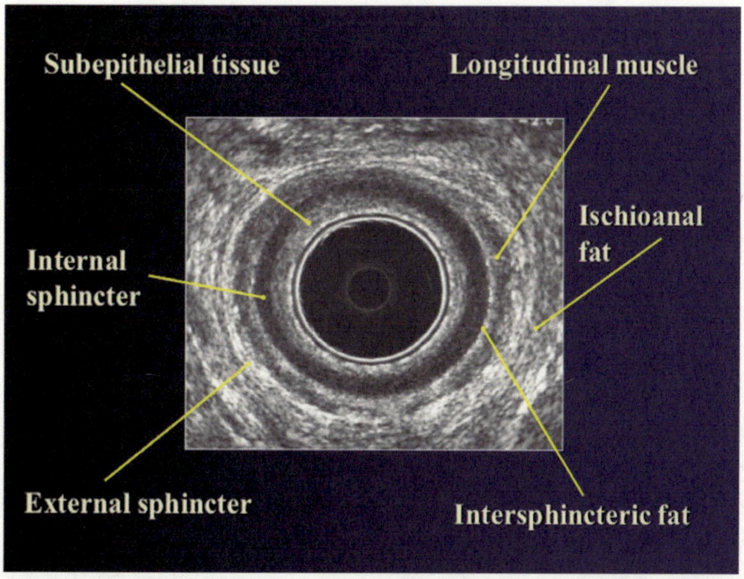

Figure 3.
Anal endoultrasonogram of a normal person. The distinct structures of the region can be seen and labeled.

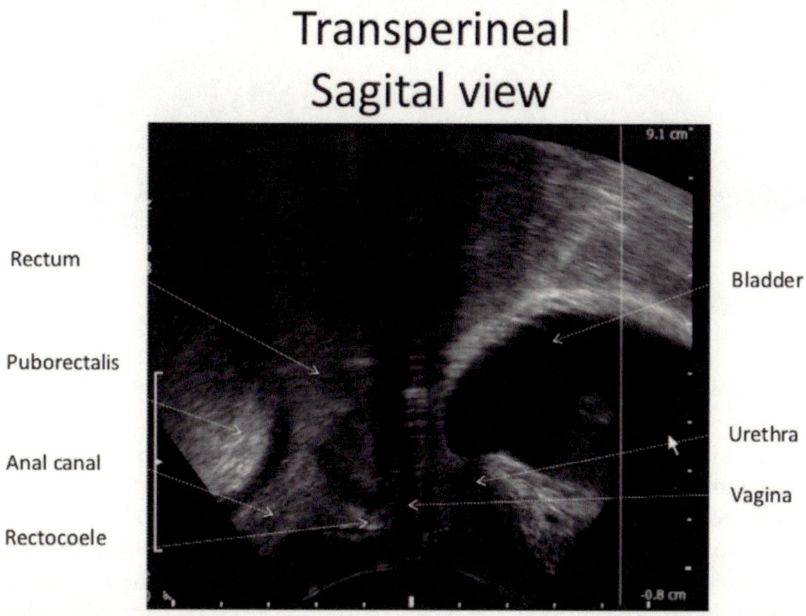

Figure 4.
Sagittal view of a transperineal ultrasonogram of a patient with rectocele, which can be discerned between the vagina and the anal canal.

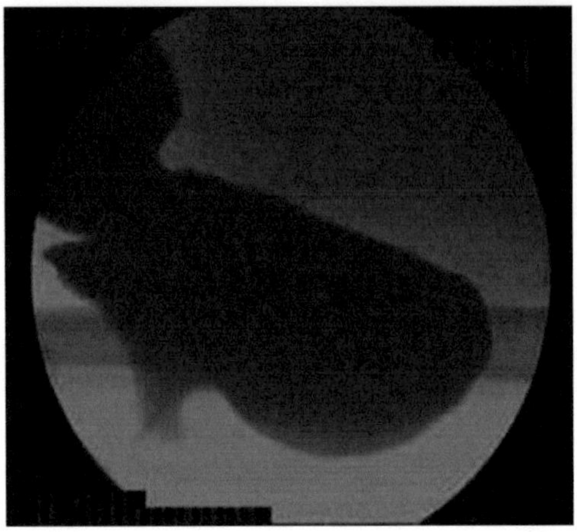

Figure 5.
Proctogram of a rectocele.

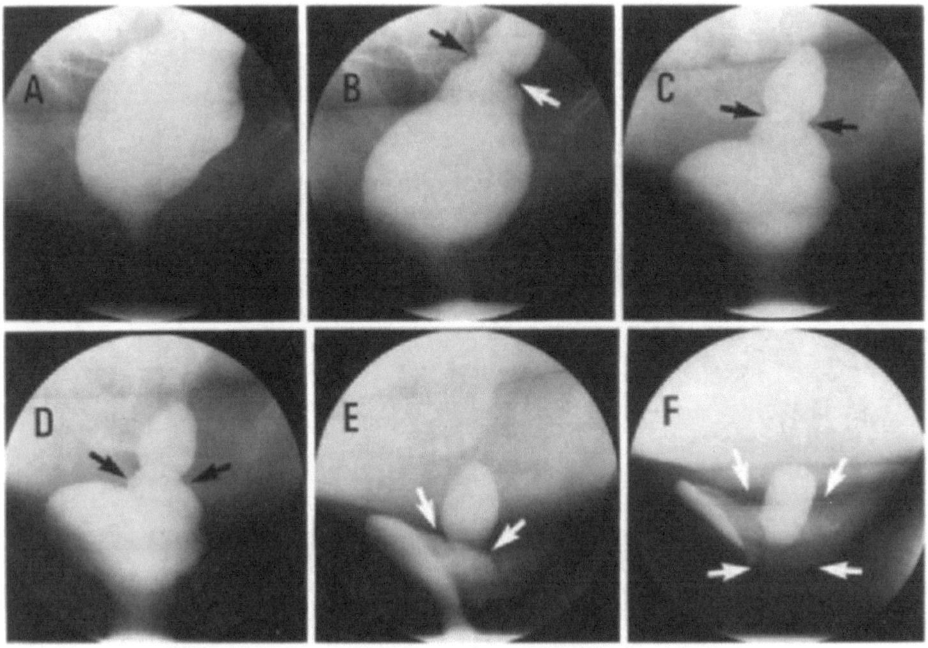

Figure 6.
Proctographic imaging of a case of anorectal intussusception.

6. Pathophysiology

As mentioned above, obstructive defecation syndrome has various clinical manifestations, but the predominant symptom is the sense of incomplete evacuation. Etiologic factors can be classified as either functional or anatomical. It is of high importance to clarify that, for patients with concomitant constipation from ODS and incontinence, soiling is coming as a result. Overlapping and mixed pathophysiology is very common. However, the most commonly accepted pathophysiological mechanisms are (a) overflow incontinence due to fecal impaction mainly in elderly people, (b) post defecation uncontrolled soiling or hard stool leakage after evacuation due to retained material, as in rectoceles, and (c) perineal denervation, pelvic floor weakness or dyssynergy which cause fecal incontinence. All of the above mechanisms are the underlying cause of obstruction defecation syndrome and contribute to fecal incontinence.

6.1 Overflow incontinence: fecal impaction

Incontinence in elder population is not uncommon. In geriatric population and particularly in institutionalized elders, prevalence of incontinence can reach 50%. Fecal impaction is defined as the prolonged retention of fecal material in the rectum. This can be a result of incomplete evacuation such as in ODS pattern, but also can happen from other causes such as immobility, hypothyroidism, neurologic disorders, dehydration, and dementia. Pharmaceutical agents such as opioids or antidepressants cause retard colonic contraction and may lead to fecal impaction. Rectum physiologically acts a fecal reservoir. Dilatation of rectal wall commences the autonomic nerve coordination for the pelvic relaxation and rectal wall contraction. In elder people, rectal sensitivity may be impaired due to chronic distention and denervation. These patients have reduced rectal sensation, pudendal neuropathy caused of chronic straining, or even concurrent reduced anal resting tone. However, when a large ball of fecal material remains for a while, secretion of mucus from rectal mucosa will cause significant soiling. Furthermore, uncontrolled contractions will end to true anal incontinence, and symptoms may be exacerbated after laxative use [17].

A similar clinical manifestation of overflow incontinence due to prolonged impaction can be seen not only in geriatric population but also in middle aged adults, although less commonly. Rectal hyposensitivity is of great importance to that type of incontinence. This is probably the underlying cause for the excessive distention of rectal wall and the development of megarectum. As a consequence, impaired rectal wall sensitivity contributes to excess rectal wall stretching and distention caused due to retained stool. As a result, paradoxical rectal contractions and overflow incontinence can happen to adult patients. In an interesting audit study from Gladman et al., rectal hyposensitivity was found in 27% of patients with coexisting constipation and incontinence [18]. On the basis of functional outlet obstruction, a few patients also have short segment Hirschsprung disease, leading to impaired rectoanal inhibitory reflex. A full rectal wall biopsy confirms the diagnosis. This disease is characterized by the absence of ganglion cells within the myenteric plexus. Rectal wall remains nonfunctional in terms of contractility, which ultimately leads to fecal retention. Surgery of the rectal wall is unusual because the same physiologic deformity usually occurs at the colonic wall. Therefore, subtotal or total colectomy is the most common surgical practice for these patients [19].

6.2 Incontinence due to rectal evacuatory disorders

As mentioned above, the most common underlying pathology of obstructive defecation syndrome is mechanical outlet obstruction. Different anatomic abnormalities can cause disruption of the normal evacuatory root. Internal rectal intussusception is probably the most common underlying pathology. It represents invagination of distal sigmoid or upper rectum to mid rectum. Traditionally, internal intussusception is considered as a precursor of true full thickness rectal prolapse and a predominant cause of ODS. It is worth to mention that intussusception is quite the common finding in proctograms. Only a minor percentage of these patients requires surgical intervention and, interestingly, many of them do not complain for clinical symptoms of ODS. Rectal prolapse occurs in only 2% of the patients with internal intussusceptions [20]. Patients suffering from years from intussusception or low take off rectal prolapse exhibit extreme straining during defecation. Eventually, this causes perineal dyssynergia from pudendal chronic neuropathy. Biofeedback remains the mainstay of treatment for this condition. The patient learns the correct technique for prompt defecation after coordination of pelvic floor muscles, under electrode monitoring [21].

Fecal incontinence in early stages of ODS is more seepage type and does not present as major episodes of leakage. It comes as an unintentional loss of small amount of liquid stool or mucus after the early hours post defecation. Patients describe a feeling of incomplete evacuation, the urge for repeated visits to toilet, incontinence or pruritus ani. Symptoms usually improve after courses of biofeedback [21]. For those who undergo surgical intervention for correction of rectoanal intussusceptions or rectocele, symptoms are also improved [22].

Apart from intussusceptions, patients with rectoceles and ODS may also have subsequent incontinence. Rectoceles can easily be detected in proctograms. These are always anterior and found only in female patients as a result of anterior herniation of rectum through the loose rectovaginal septum, causing bulging of posterior vaginal wall. Again, as in intussusception, rectocele may represent only a radiological finding in asymptomatic women. Biofeedback remains the cornerstone of the treatment algorithm. Small rectoceles usually do not require surgical intervention. Incontinence symptoms improve postoperatively in patients who are submitted to operation. Laparoscopic ventral mesh rectopexy has become the treatment of choice for fit female patients, mainly in Europe [23]. Perineal or transvaginal rectocele repair with or without levatorplasty is another option, with promising results in experienced centers [24]. Stapled transanal rectal resection procedure (STARR/TRANSTARR) has gained a wide acceptance among colorectal surgeons. The concept is the removal of the redundant anterior or circumferential rectal mucosa, allowing a straightened outlet [25, 26].

Although surgery for ODS has gained great acceptance between colorectal surgeons, it is crucial to understand that it is needed only for correction of major anatomic abnormalities. Furthermore, surgery for ODS may aggravate any symptoms of urgency, as well as cause subsequent incontinence, thus it is not without pitfalls or risks. Among the different techniques available for fixing rectoceles or intussusception, laparoscopic ventral mesh rectopexy seems to have the less risk of postoperative incontinence. However, it requires expert knowledge of the technique, its results are not widely reproducible, and mesh complications may lead surgeons to abandon the technique in the future [27, 28]. The Delorme and the Internal Delorme procedures have been widely used for rectal prolapse and for low take off prolapse or intussusception respectively, as causes of ODS symptoms. Internal mucosa excision and plication completely restores the rectal cavity, reducing, however, in the process, the rectal capacity and compliance. The resulting rectal hyposensitivity and abnormal distention contribute to urge incontinence. For patients with preoperative anal incontinence and rectal prolapse Delorme or Internal Delorme procedures should be avoided [29, 30] Regarding the STARR technique, which is widely used to correct both rectocele and intussusception, criticism has been raised due to the lack of long-term results, as well as the worsening of urge incontinence in some patients. An Italian study on patients who underwent STARR reported increased predominantly incidence of urge type of incontinence. Maximum tolerated rectal volume capacity was impaired according to anorectal manometry [31]. The European Stapled Transanal Rectal Resection Registry reports urgency in about 20% of operated patients. Impaired rectal compliance and even minimal sphincter damage from the stapler can easily transform defecatory urgency to urge fecal incontinence [32].

6.3 Incontinence due to dyssynergia and pelvic floor weakness

Dyssynergia, by all means, is a syndrome of different specific origins, with symptoms that can be produced by lack of coordination or malfunction of different pelvic muscles. Thus, pelvic dyssynergia generally results from paradoxic muscle spasm and failure of puborectalis sling to relax during defecation. As a consequence, functional outlet obstruction is not unusual. Rectal masses should be excluded with flexible sigmoidoscopy at the first instance and anatomic abnormalities as intussusception and rectoceles should be excluded—usually with a proctogram. Defecography is also crucial to recognize anismic patients and paradoxic spasm of the puborectalis muscle. Anal manometry usually shows increased anal rest pressures, failure of relaxation, and increased puborectalis activity during straining [16]. In proctograms, anorectal angle changes less than 15°, and the perineum fails to relax and to descend during defecation. There are different studies that show the connection between dyssynergia and fecal seepage or soiling. In the study of Rao SS et al., in 25 patients who reported seepage, residual anal pressure was raised and 29% were unable to expel a rectal balloon [33]. As mentioned above, rectal sensation is crucial, thus rectal hyposensitivity, which is common in functional obstruction syndrome, results in impaired rectoanal coordination and pelvic muscles relaxation.

Biofeedback is the first step in the treatment of patient with ODS and is mainly useful for patients with pelvic floor dyssynergy. It is a sophisticated approach using behavioral and physiologic methods. Biofeedback uses anorectal manometers and screen in front of the patient, where changes in attempts for defecation and correction of the technique can be visible for the patient, recognizing different patterns of muscular activity. The majority of patients report improved outcomes after repeated courses of biofeedback. For patients with rectal intussusception and small rectoceles, this is the treatment of choice [21]. Botulinum toxin injection is another option for anismic patients. Injection of 60–100 U on the puborectalis sling showed prominent results in patients with pelvic dyssynergy, although the lack of long-term data and the need for repeated injections [34].

The role of SNS in obstructive defecation has been debatable. Most of the studies for SNS have been done for patients with slow transit constipation or incontinence, and few data are available for ODS. Some of these patients report improvement of straining, but still more studies are required [35].

Pelvic floor weakness and pudendal denervation due to chronic straining or repeated perineum stretching had been traditionally considered as the principal mechanism for fecal incontinence. Prolonged straining, descent of perineum, and prolapse cause not only anal sphincter disruption but also chronic pudendal neuropathy. As a result, anal pressures are reduced and this predisposes to incontinence [36]. Pudendal neuropathy needs time to be established, but time is crucial because once it is established, the malfunction becomes permanent. In a longitudinal study of patients with perineal descending syndrome, more than 50% became incontinent in a second follow up 5 years after initial assessment [37]. In general, pelvic floor weakness, with all clinical presentations (rectocele, descending perineum, prolapsed) and organ prolapse predispose to evacuatory disorders and denervation, causing finally fecal incontinence.

7. Conclusions

Fecal incontinence is a quite common and underestimated clinical syndrome, which is not exclusive to aged patients. Great clinical expertise is needed for the assessment of the patients. Obstructive defecation syndrome has been nowadays accepted as one of the underlying pathologies that ultimately lead to fecal incontinence. Clinical assessment, defecatory proctogram, anorectal manometry evaluation, and endoanal ultrasound are the tools needed for a full discussion on a pelvic floor MDT. Conservative management with biofeedback is a key to the treatment, and of great benefit to the patients. Surgery for ODS should be offered only to patients who fail biofeedback or have major anatomic abnormalities. The decision of the type of surgery that will be suggested to the patient must be decided after a great deal of thought, because different procedures for ODS may lead to fecal incontinence as well.

Acknowledgements

The author would like to acknowledge the work of Dr. Spyridon Smparounis in proofreading and correcting the drafts of this manuscript.

Author details

Dimitrios Linardoutsos
Advanced Laparoscopic Department of Surgery, Metropolitan General Hospital, Cholargos, Athens, Greece

*Address all correspondence to: dlinardoutsos@gmail.com

References

[1] Fritsch H et al. Clinical anatomy of the pelvic floor. Advances in Anatomy, Embryology, and Cell Biology. 2004;**175**:1-64

[2] Vrees MD, Weiss EG. The evaluation of constipation. Clinics in Colon and Rectal Surgery. 2005;**18**(2):65-75

[3] Barrett J, Kiff E, et al. Anorectal function in the elderly. In: Coloproctology and the Pelvic Floor. 2nd ed. Oxford: Butterworth-Heinemann Ltd; 1992. pp. 470-476

[4] Chatoor DR, Taylor SJ, et al. Fecal incontinence. The British Journal of Surgery. 2007;**94**(2):134-144

[5] Snooks SJ, Barnes PR, et al. Damage to the innervation of the pelvic floor musculature in chronic constipation. Gastroenterology. 1985;**89**(5):977-981

[6] Wald A. Clinical practise. Fecal incontinence in adults. The New England Journal of Medicine. 2007;**356**(16):1648-1655

[7] Whitehead WE, Borrud L, et al. Fecal incontinence in US adults: Epidemiology and risk factors. Gastroenterology. 2009;**137**(2):512-517

[8] Scott SM, Luniss PJ, Ratto C, Doglietto GB, editors. Risk factors in faecal incontinence. In: Faecal Incontinence. Diagnosis and Treatment. London UK: Springer-Verlag London Ltd; 2007. pp. 43-66

[9] Damon H, Guye O, et al. Prevalence of anal incontinence in adults and impact and impact on quality of life. Gastroentérologie Clinique et Biologique. 2006;**30**(1):37-43

[10] Bharucha AE, Zinsmeister AR, et al. Bowel disturbances are the most important risk factors for late onset fecal incontinence: A population-based case-control study in women. Gastroenterology;**139**(5):Q1559-Q1566

[11] Bener A, Saleh N, et al. Prevalence and determinants of fecal incontinence in premenopausal women in Arabian community. Climacteric. 2008;**11**(5):429-435

[12] Rex DK, Lappas JC. Combined anorectal manometry and defecography in 50 consecutive adults with fecal incontinence. Diseases of the Colon and Rectum. 1992;**35**(11):1040-1045

[13] Harewood GC, Coulie B, Camilleri M, Rath-Harvey D, et al. Descending perineum syndrome: Audit of clinical and laboratory features and outcome of pelvic floor retraining. The American Journal of Gastroenterology. 1999;**94**(1):126-130

[14] Mohamed SD. Co-existence of constipation and faecal incontinence: A greatly underappreciated clinical problem. Neurogastroenterology and Motility. 2010;**22**:37

[15] Burgell RE. Fecal incontinence in men: Coexistent constipation and impact of real hyposensitivity. Gastroenterology. 2010;**138**:542

[16] Videlock EJ, Lembo A, Cremonini F. Diagnostic testing for dyssynergic defecation in chronic constipation: Meta-analysis. Neurogastroenterology and Motility. 2013;**25**(6):509-520

[17] Cooper ZR, Rose S. Fecal incontinence: A clinical approach. Mount Sinai Journal of Medicine. 2000;**67**(2):96-105

[18] Gladman MA, Luniss PJ, et al. Rectal hyposensivity. The American Journal of Gastroenterology. 2006;**101**(5):1140-1151

[19] Parisi MA. Hirshprung disease overview. Current Opinion in Pediatrics. 2000;**12**(6):610-617

[20] Siproudhis L, Pigot F, Godeberge P, Damon H, Soudan D, Bigard MA. Defecation disorders: A French population survey. Diseases of the Colon and Rectum. 2006;**49**(2):219-227

[21] Rao SS, Valestin J, Brown CK, Zimmerman B, Schulze K. Long-term efficacy of biofeedback therapy for dyssynergic defecation: Randomized controlled trial. The American Journal of Gastroenterology. 2010;**105**(4):890-896

[22] Mercer-Jones MA, D'Hoore A, Dixon AR, Lehur P, Lindsey I, Mellgren A, et al. Consensus on ventral rectopexy: Report of a panel of experts. Colorectal Disease. 2014;**16**(2):82-88

[23] D'Hoore A, Penninckx F. Laparoscopic ventral recto(colpo)pexy for rectal prolapse: Surgical technique and outcome for 109 patients. Surgical Endoscopy. 2006;**20**(12):1919-1923

[24] Lehur PA, Stuto A, Fantoli M, Villani RD, Queralto M, Lazorthes F, et al. ODS II Study Group. Outcomes of stapled transanal rectal resection vs. biofeedback for the treatment of outlet obstruction associated with rectal intussusception and rectocele: A multicenter, randomized, controlled trial. Diseases of the Colon and Rectum. 2008;**51**(11):1611-1618

[25] Van Geluwe B, Stuto A, Da Pozzo F, Fieuws S, Meurette G, Lehur PA, et al. Relief of obstructed defecation syndrome after stapled transanal rectal resection (STARR): A meta-analysis. Acta Chirurgica Belgica. 2014;**114**(3):189-197

[26] Ribaric G, D'Hoore A, Schiffhorst G, Hempel E. TRANSTAR Registry Study Group. STARR with CONTOUR® TRANSTAR™ device for obstructed defecation syndrome: One-year real-world outcomes of the European TRANSTAR registry. International Journal of Colorectal Disease. 2014;**29**(5):611-622

[27] Ahmad NZ, Stefan S, et al. Laparoscopic ventral mesh rectopexy: Functional outcomes after surgery. Journal of Surgery. 2018;**4**(4):e205-e211

[28] Borie F, Coste T, et al. Incidence and surgical treatment of synthetic mesh-related infectious complications after laparoscopic ventral rectopexy. Techniques in Coloproctology. 2016;**20**(11):759-765

[29] Emile SH, Elbanna H, et al. Laparoscopic ventral mesh rectopexy vs Delorme's operation in management of complete rectal prolapse: A prospective randomised study. Colorectal Disease. 2017;**19**:50-57

[30] Cavazzoni E, Rosati E, et al. Simultaneous Delorme's procedure and inter-sphincteric prosthetic implant for the treatment of rectal prolapse and faecal incontinence: Preliminary experience and literature review. International Journal of Surgery. 2015;**14**:45-48

[31] Pucciani F. Post-surgical fecal incontinence. Updates in Surgery. 2018;**70**(4):477-484

[32] Jayne DG, Schwander O, et al. Stapled transanal rectal resection for obstructed defecation syndrome: One-year results of the european STARR registry. Diseases of the Colon and Rectum;**52**:1205-1212

[33] Rao SS, Ozturk R, et al. Investigation of the pathophysiology of fecal seapage. The American Journal of Gastroenterology. 2004;**99**(11):2204-2209

[34] Hompes R, Harmston C, et al. Excellent response rate of anismus to botulinum toxin if rectal prolapsed misdiagnosed as anismus (pseudoanismus) is excluded. Colorectal Disease. 2012;**14**(2):224-230

[35] Ganio E, Masin A, et al. Short term sacral nerve stimulation for functional anorectal and urinary disturbances: Results in 40 patients: Evaluation of a new option for anorectal functional disorders. Diseases of the Colon and Rectum. 2001;**44**(9):1261-1267

[36] Kiff ES, Barnes PR, et al. Evidence of pudendal neuropathy in patients with perineal descent and chronic straining at stool. Gut. 1984;**25**(11):1279-1282

[37] Berkelmans I, Heresbach D, et al. Perineal descent at defecography in women with straining at stool: A lack of specificity or predictive value for future anal incontinence? European Journal of Gastroenterology & Hepatology. 1995;**7**(1):75-79

Section 4

Faecal Incontinence and Systemic Disease

Chapter 5

Faecal Incontinence and Autoimmune Diseases

Batool Mutar Mahdi

Abstract

Anal and rectal continence depend on many factors such as such as consistency of stool, integrity of neuromuscular sphincter complex, rectal capacity, sensation of defecation, higher cerebral function, and mobility. Any disturbance to these parameters may lead to various degrees of faecal incontinence. Continence may also be affected by immunological disorders that cause vasculitis as well as gastrointestinal mucosal and smooth muscle damage due to the formation of autoantibodies and immune complexes in autoimmune disease. A thorough knowledge of the gastrointestinal manifestations of autoimmune disease is important in order to be able to manage patients' symptoms optimally.

Keywords: autoimmunity, immune tolerance, inflammasomes, cytokines, faecal incontinence

1. Introduction

Faecal incontinence is characterized by inability to control bowel motions, causing the unexpected leakage of flatus and feces per rectum [1]. It may adversely affect the quality of one's life. Faecal incontinence may be precipitated by conditions such as diarrhea, constipation, pelvic muscle damage, nerve damage, and vaginal delivery. Faecal continence depends on many factors; for example, consistency of faecal substance, neuromuscular sphincter complex, rectal capacity, and sensation of defecation [2]. Other causes of faecal incontinence include immunological disorders that cause muscle damage due to formation of autoantibodies in autoimmune diseases [3, 4].

2. What is autoimmunity?

Autoimmunity is a disorder of the immune system. It is characterised by the absence of immune tolerance (tolerance is the absence of an immune response in an immunologically competent person), be it central tolerance in the thymus or peripheral tolerance through Treg cell CD4+ and CD25+ (T regularity). It is due to a defect in immune regulatory and signaling mechanisms; genetic factors like single-gene defects or gene mutation can also cause an immune dysregulation and autoimmunity [5].

3. Causes of autoimmunity

3.1 Epigenetic alterations

Epigenetic alterations like DNA methylation, histone modification, and microRNAs alter the transcription and activity of genes that are involved in autoimmune responses and disease pathogenesis. These lead to aberrant epigenetic modifications in CD4 T helper cells' function through deregulations in several transcriptional genes like Ifng, Cd70, Tnf, Dnmt3a, and Foxp3 that determine T cell identity. Adding to this, epigenetics target regulatory genes like Tim-3, cereblon, protein kinase C theta, octamer transcription factor 1, basic leucine zipper transcription factor ATF-like, p70 kinase, and lactate dehydrogenase A that influence T cell activation, differentiation, and metabolism [6].

3.2 Genetic mutation in inflammasome

Inflammasomes are multi-protein complexes that consist of NOD-like receptor (NLR) and AIM-like receptor (ALR) and apoptosis-associated speck-like protein that contains a CARD and caspase-1. The active caspase-1 cleaves pro-IL-1β and pro-IL-18 to IL-1β and IL-18, resulting in inflammation. Genetic mutations in inflammasomes result in autoimmune diseases. NOD-like receptor family, pyrin domain containing 1 (NLRP1) haplotypes contributes to susceptibility to autoimmune disease and single nucleotide polymorphisms (SNPs) that alter the susceptibility and severity of autoimmune disease. IL-1β and IL-18 maintain Th17 responses and endothelial cell damage, which potentiate autoimmune diseases. Autoimmunity is mediated in part by innocent bystander cells, augmented by inflammasomes [7].

3.3 HLA-associated autoimmune diseases

Autoimmune diseases have associations with particular HLA alleles through displaying the autoantigens targeted by self-reactive T cells that escape thymic deletion because most HLA alleles are capable of presenting self-antigens even in healthy individuals [8].

3.4 Cytokines pathway

Cytokine and cytokine receptor genetic polymorphisms have been associated with many different autoimmune diseases like *IL23R* and IL-23 that augment the pro-inflammatory action of Th17 cells that leads to tissue damage, and anti-cytokine therapy can be nicely used as a target to treat autoimmune diseases [9–11].

4. Mechanism of autoimmunity

The mechanism of autoimmune reactions is due to an imbalance between two immune responses, effector and regulatory, that develop through stages of initiation and propagation, and often show phases of resolution or remissions and exacerbations or flares. The mechanism of autoimmunity is defective elimination and/or control of self-reactive lymphocytes. A major goal of treatment is reestablishing the normal balance between effector and regulatory immune responses [12] (**Figure 1**).

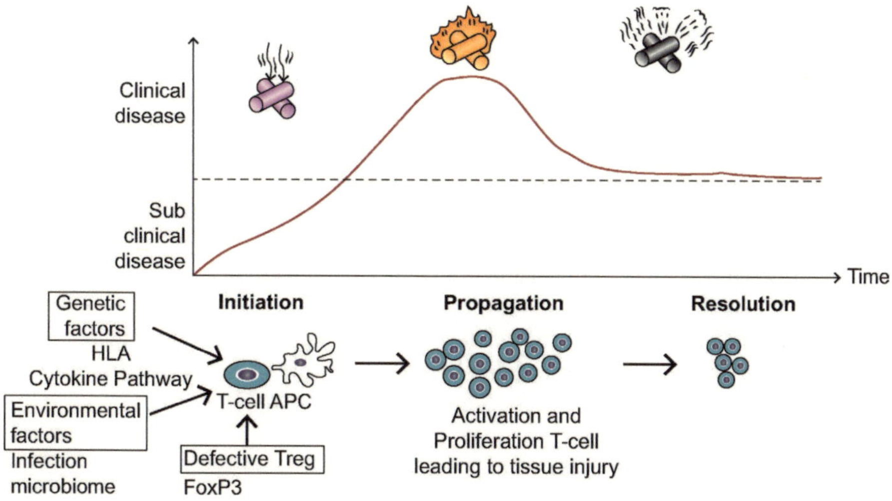

Figure 1.
Mechanism of autoimmunity.

5. Gastrointestinal manifestations in systemic autoimmune diseases

The systemic autoimmune diseases include different diseases like collagen vascular diseases, systemic vasculitides, Wegener granulomatosis, and Churg-Strauss syndrome that involve any part of gastrointestinal tract, hepatobiliary system, and pancreas. Patients with these diseases had different gastrointestinal symptoms like oral ulcers, dysphagia, gastroesophageal reflux diseases, abdominal pain, constipation, diarrhea, faecal incontinence, pseudo-obstruction, perforation of GIT tract, and bleeding [13].

5.1 Effects of autoimmune diseases on the gastrointestinal tract

Some autoimmune diseases are characterized by autoreactive T cells attacking body's own tissues. One of the manifestations of these diseases is gastrointestinal manifestation, which is either the initial presentation or the complications of the disease.

5.1.1 Systemic lupus erythematosus

Systemic lupus erythematosus (SLE) is an autoimmune disease of unknown etiology, characterized by deposition of autoantibodies and immune complexes in tissues (type III hypersensitivity). Gastrointestinal manifestations of SLE are due to primary gastrointestinal disorders, complications of therapy, and SLE itself. Any part of the gastrointestinal tract may become involved in SLE. Many GI conditions can be mimicked by SLE [14]. Lupus enteritis, a distinct subset of SLE, is defined as either vasculitis or inflammation of the small bowel. The clinical manifestations include decreased salivation, buccal mucosal ulcers, dysphagia, oesophageal ulceration, gastric ulceration, pseudo-obstruction, and faecal incontinence [15–17].

5.1.2 Rheumatoid arthritis

It is also a type III hyper sensitivity reaction due to deposition of immune complexes in the synovium of small interphalangeal joints of hands. Gastrointestinal manifestations are common and variable. It involves the esophagus resulting in decreased peristalsis, decreased lower esophageal sphincter tone, hiatal hernia, and esophageal ulcer. It may also result in peptic ulcer and chronic atrophic gastritis. Colonic inflammation such as collagenous colitis with secondary amyloidosis may also occur, leading to diarrhea and faecal incontinence [18].

5.1.3 Sjogren's syndrome

Sjögren syndrome is a common autoimmune disease due to B cell activation and invasion of T and B lymphocytes to affected exocrine glands. This disease affects the gastrointestinal tract resulting in dry mouth, difficulty in swallowing, esophageal atrophy, epigastric pain, dyspepsia, chronic atrophic gastritis, chronic pancreatitis, jejunitis, sigmoiditis, and inflammatory bowel disease [19, 20].

5.1.4 Progressive systemic sclerosis (scleroderma)

It is one of the connective tissue diseases of unknown etiology that affects females more than males. It is characterized by vasculopathy, tissue fibrosis, and autoimmunity. It causes overproduction of collagen due to autoimmune dysfunction that leads to fibrosis of many visceral organs. The immune system attacks the kinetochore of the chromosomes that leads to genetic malformation of nearby genes. Patients experience gastrointestinal tract symptoms like thinning of the lips, tightening of the perioral skin, impaired taste sensation, atrophy of the mucous membrane and tongue papilla, dysphagia and dyspepsia, gastroesophageal reflux, peptic esophagitis, Barrett's metaplasia, gastric antral vascular ectasia (GAVE) or watermelon stomach, and dysmotility of small intestine leading to chronic pseudo-obstruction. As scleroderma progresses, it may lead to decreased motility of the intestine and to progressive fibrosis and scarring of the small intestine leading to bacterial overgrowth and malabsorption of nutrients and growth in stagnant intestinal fluid. Large intestine and colon will be involved, causing pseudo-obstruction or ischemic colitis [21, 22]. Anorectal involvement causes faecal incontinence and rectal prolapse. Gastrointestinal tract involvement greatly affects morbidity and mortality in this disease and therapy aims to relieve these symptoms [23, 24].

5.1.5 Polyarteritis nodosa

The gastrointestinal manifestations of systemic vasculitis that results from mesenteric ischemia are vague nonspecific abdominal pain, hematemesis, melena, hematochezia, jejunal ulceration, and perforation. Liver may be involved with acalculous cholecystitis, appendicitis, pancreatitis, and biliary strictures [25–27].

5.1.6 Kawasaki disease

This is a syndrome that is characterized by oral mucosal changes, fever, lymphadenopathy, and polyarteritis in addition to gastrointestinal symptoms like abdominal pain, vomiting, diarrhea, small bowel obstruction, jaundice, and paralytic ileus [28].

5.1.7 Inflammatory muscle disorders: polymyositis and dermatomyositis

These are systemic autoimmune diseases characterized by inflammation of striated and smooth muscle of the body. Patients had a progressive weakness of proximal striated muscles and skin rash with dermatomyositis. The whole gastrointestinal tract may be affected but the proximal esophagus is more common affected. Gastric and esophageal emptying and peristalsis are affected in many patients, so they complain of dysphagia, aspiration, nasal regurgitation, early satiety, bloating, reduced gastrointestinal motility, hiatal hernia, gastroesophageal reflux disease (GERD), stricture, dilated atonic esophagus associated with delayed gastric emptying, and intestinal mucosal thickening. In addition to that, there are colonic pseudodiverticulosis and pneumatosis coli. Neurological dysfunction and diminished smooth muscle contractility due to muscle atrophy and fibrosis lead to bowel wall oedema, ulceration, and perforation [29].

5.1.8 Giant cell arteritis

This is a granulomatous inflammation of the arteries, particularly cranial and temporal, leading to narrowing the lumen of the arteries. The main symptoms are headache and fever. Blindness may occur suddenly. There are associations with intestinal manifestations like bowel ischemia and gangrene, acute pancreatitis, liver granulomas, lymphocytic infiltration, and dilated bile canaliculi. The erythrocyte sedimentation rate is high [30, 31].

5.1.9 Henoch-Schönlein purpura

This is an IgA-mediated immune complex deposit resulting in systemic vasculitis in small vessels. Gastrointestinal signs and symptoms are common such as periumbilical pain with nausea and vomiting. Sometimes ulceration of the mucosa of the second part of the duodenum and less commonly in the colon and rectum may occur [32].

5.1.10 Takayasu arteritis

This is a chronic vasculitis of unknown etiology. The inflammatory processes cause thickening, narrowing, and eventual occlusion of the walls of the affected arteries. Patients usually experience gastrointestinal symptoms such as abdominal pain, nausea, diarrhea, and hemorrhage due to the involvement of the descending abdominal aorta [33].

5.1.11 Cogan's syndrome

This is a chronic inflammatory disorder characterized by interstitial keratitis, audiovestibular system involvement, aortitis, mesenteric vasculitis, weight loss, fever, lymphadenopathy, hepatosplenomegaly, abdominal pain, nausea, and vomiting [34].

5.1.12 Churg-Strauss syndrome

This is an allergic angiitis that occurs mostly in asthmatic patients, and is associated with granulomatous necrotizing vasculitis. Patients have eosinophilia, fever, and allergic rhinitis. Sometimes gastrointestinal involvement occurs in about 50% of patients, leading to eosinophilic gastroenteritis associated with abdominal pain, bloody diarrhea due to multiple ulcers, nausea, and vomiting. Perforation of the small intestine and colon may commonly occur. Necrotizing granulomatous vasculitis of the mesenteric artery leads to mucosal ischemia [35].

5.1.13 Wegener granulomatosis

This is a systemic autoimmune disease characterized by granulomatous vasculitis of the upper and lower respiratory tracts leading to infection, glomerulonephritis, and small-vessel necrotizing vasculitis with granuloma formation. Gastrointestinal manifestations of Wegener granulomatosis are oropharyngeal mucosal lesions, gingivitis, ulcer of gastric mucosa, small intestinal perforation, colonic ulceration, non-healing perianal ulcers, cholecystitis, recurrent acute pancreatitis, and splenic necrosis [25].

5.1.14 Antiphospholipid antibody syndrome

This is a disorder characterized by recurrent vascular thrombosis, abortion, and thrombocytopenia due to increased antiphospholipid antibodies. The gastrointestinal manifestations of antiphospholipid antibody syndrome lead to vasculopathy and tissue ischemia. Antiphospholipid antibodies in SLE patients are associated with Budd-Chiari syndrome, with patients presenting with abdominal pain, ascites, and hepatic failure [36–38].

5.1.15 Spondyloarthropathies

These are a group of interconnected chronic inflammatory rheumatic diseases including ankylosing spondylitis, arthritis associated with inflammatory bowel disease and reactive arthritis. The spondyloarthropathies are associated with the HLA-B27 gene. About 36% of patients have reactive arthritis secondary to a dysenteric infection were positive for HLA-B27. Subclinical gut inflammation, ulcerative colitis, and Crohn's disease are frequent types of idiopathic IBD that are associated with arthritis or spondylitis [39–43].

5.1.16 Behçet's disease

This is a widespread autoimmune vasculitis of unknown origin occurring in all ages resulting in a damage to blood vessels in all the body. Patients usually had uveitis with oral and genital ulcers. Clinical manifestations also include vascular, neurological, articular, renal, and gastrointestinal manifestations. Gastrointestinal Behçet's disease symptoms are similar to those caused by inflammatory bowel diseases, and include nausea, abdominal pain, and bloody diarrhea. In addition, ulceration in the mouth, gastrointestinal tract, or genitalia may occur, the ulcers typically being painful, shallow and round with discrete borders. Segmental mucosal ulceration in the ileocecal and colonic area leads to perforation and bloody diarrhea [44].

6. Mechanisms of how autoimmune disorders cause faecal incontinence

The precise cause and mechanism how autoimmune diseases cause faecal incontinence are unknown, but multiple factors are probably involved. These factors include deterioration and destruction of collagen framework by the effect of autoantibodies, resulting in inflammation, reduced compliance of rectal muscles with consequent urgency, and urge faecal incontinence. Diarrhea is one of GIT manifestation of autoimmune connective tissue diseases, and this in itself may lead to incontinence even in the presence of normal sphincters.

DOI: http://dx.doi.org/10.5772/intechopen.89290

7. Conclusion

Continence usually requires normal functioning of both the muscles of the lower digestive tract and pelvic floor, and the nervous system. There are many causes of faecal incontinence. In this chapter, we have discussed the various autoimmune disorders and their involvement in the disruption of the continence mechanism. Further studies are necessary in this field, focusing on targeted therapies to minimize the effect of these diseases on the gastrointestinal tract.

Author details

Batool Mutar Mahdi
HLA Research Unit, Department of Microbiology, Al-Kindy College of Medicine, University of Baghdad, Baghdad, Iraq

*Address all correspondence to: abas_susan@yahoo.com

References

[1] Ditah I, Devaki P, Luma HN, Ditah C, Njei B, Jaiyeoba C, et al. Prevalence, trends, and risk factors for fecal incontinence in United States adults, 2005-2010. Clinical Gastroenterology and Hepatology. 2014;**12**:636-643.e2

[2] Landenfeld CS, Bowers BJ, Feld AD, Hartmann KE, Hoffman E, Ingber MJ, et al. National Institutes of Health State-of-the-Science Conference statement: Prevention of fecal and urinary incontinence in adults. Annals of Internal Medicine. 2008;**148**:449-458

[3] Chirkin VV, Martynova TI, Dul'tsev IV. Immunological disorders and their correction in patients with incompetence of the anal sphincter. Khirurgiia (Mosk). 1983;**3**:88-92

[4] Coura MM, Silva SM, Almeida RM, Forrest MC, Sousa JB. Is digital rectal exam reliable in grading anal sphincter defects? Arquivos de Gastroenterologia. 2016;**53**:240-245

[5] Schmidt RE, Grimbacher B, Witte T. Autoimmunity and primary immunodeficiency: Two sides of the same coin? Nature Reviews Rheumatology. 2017;**14**:7-18

[6] Wang Z, Chang C, Lu Q. Epigenetics of CD4+ T cells in autoimmune diseases. Current Opinion in Rheumatology. 2017;**29**:361-368

[7] Yang CA, Chiang BL. Inflammasomes and human autoimmunity: A comprehensive review. Journal of Autoimmunity. 2015;**61**:1-8

[8] Goris A, Liston A. The immunogenetic architecture of autoimmune disease. Cold Spring Harbor Perspectives in Biology. 2012;**4**:a007260

[9] Ghoreschi K et al. Generation of pathogenic T(H)17 cells in the absence of TGF-β signalling. Nature. 2010;**467**(7318):967-971

[10] Vandenbroeck K. Cytokine gene polymorphisms and human autoimmune disease in the era of genome-wide association studies. Journal of Interferon & Cytokine Research. 2012;**32**:139-151

[11] Elliott M et al. Ustekinumab: Lessons learned from targeting interleukin-12/23p40 in immune-mediated diseases. Annals of the New York Academy of Sciences. 2009;**1182**:97-110

[12] Rosenblum MD, Remedios KA, Abbas AK. Mechanisms of human autoimmunity. The Journal of Clinical Investigation. 2015;**125**:2228-2233

[13] Cojocaru M, Cojocaru IM, Silosi I, Vrabie CD. Gastrointestinal manifestations in systemic autoimmune diseases. Maedica (Buchar). 2011;**6**:45-51

[14] Rich RR, Fleisher TA, Shearer WT, et al. Clinical Immunology. Principles and Practice. 2nd ed. London: Mosby International Limited; 2001

[15] Mok MY, Wong RWS, Lau CS. Intestinal pseudo-obstruction in systemic lupus erythematosus an uncommon but important clinical manifestation. Lupus. 2000;**9**:11-18

[16] Tian X-P, Zhang X. Gastrointestinal involvement in systemic lupus erythematosus: Insight into pathogenesis, diagnosis and treatment. World Journal of Gastroenterology. 2010;**16**:2971-2977

[17] Alves SC, Fasano S, Isenberg DA. Autoimmune gastrointestinal complications in patients with systemic lupus erythematosus: Case

series and literature review. Lupus. 2016;**25**:1509-1519

[18] Wordsworth P. Arthritis and inflammatory bowel disease. Current Rheumatology Reports. 2000;**2**:87-88

[19] Shahzad HS, Shaw-Stiffel TA. The gastrointestinal manifestations of Sjögren's syndrome. The American Journal of Gastroenterology. 1995;**90**:9-14

[20] Popov Y, Salomon-Escoto K. Gastrointestinal and hepatic disease in Sjogren syndrome. Rheumatic Diseases Clinics of North America. 2018;**44**:143-151

[21] Ponge T, Bruley des Varannes S. Digestive involvement of scleroderma. La Revue du Praticien. 2002;**52**: 1896-1900

[22] Sallam H, McNearney TA, Chen JD. Systematic review: Pathophysiology and management of gastrointestinal dysmotility in systemic sclerosis (scleroderma). Alimentary Pharmacology & Therapeutics. 2006;**23**:601-712

[23] Marie I. Gastrointestinal involvement in systemic sclerosis. Presse Médicale. 2006;**35**:1952-1965

[24] Stelle M, Chizzolini C. Gastrointestinal features in systemic sclerosis. Revue Médicale Suisse. 2014;**10**:860-863

[25] Pagnoux C, Mahr A, Cohen P, et al. Presentation and outcome of gastrointestinal involvement in systemic necrotizing vasculitides: Analysis of 62 patients with polyarteritis nodosa, microscopic polyangiitis, Wegener granulomatosis, Churg-Strauss syndrome, or rheumatoid arthritis-associated vasculitis. Medicine (Baltimore). 2005;**84**:115-128

[26] Levine SM, Hellmann DB, Stone JH. Gastrointestinal involvement in polyarteritis nodosa (1986-2000): Presentation and outcomes in 24 patients. The American Journal of Medicine. 2002;**112**:386-391

[27] Ebert EC, Hagspiel KD, Nagar M, et al. Gastrointestinal involvement in polyarteritis nodosa. Clinical Gastroenterology and Hepatology. 2008;**6**:960-966

[28] Chen WT, Huang SR, Wang JK. Kawasaki disease presenting with hepatitis and prolonged fever. Report of one case. Acta Paediatrica Taiwanica. 2003;**44**:174-176

[29] Ebert EC. Review article: The gastrointestinal complications of myositis. Alimentary Pharmacology & Therapeutics. 2010;**31**:359-365

[30] Annamalai A, Francis ML, Ranatunga SKM, et al. Giant cell arteritis presenting as small bowel infaction. Journal of General Internal Medicine. 2007;**22**:140-144

[31] Trimble MA, Weisz MA. Infarction of the sigmoid colon secondary to giant cell arteritis. Rheumatology (Oxford, England). 2002;**41**:108-110

[32] Chang W-L, Yang Y-H, Lin Y-T, et al. Gastrointestinal manifestations in Henoch-Schönlein purpura: A review of 261 patients. Acta Paediatrica. 2004;**93**:1427-1431

[33] Zamani F, Shakeri R, Modiramani O, et al. Medscape General Medicine. 2006;**8**:69

[34] Gluth MB, Baratz KH, Matteson EL, et al. Cogan syndrome: A retrospective review of 60 patients throughout a half century. Mayo Clinic Proceedings. 2006;**81**:483-488

[35] Vaglio A, Corradi D, Ronda N, et al. Large bowel obstruction heralding Churg-Strauss syndrome. The American Journal of Gastroenterology. 2004;**99**:562-563

[36] Braham A, Safer L, Bdioui F, et al. Antiphospholipid antibodies in digestive diseases. Presse Médicale. 2001;**30**:1890-1897

[37] Asherson RA, Cervera R. Unusual manifestations of the antiphospholipid syndrome. Clinical Reviews in Allergy and Immunology. 2003;**25**:61-78

[38] Spencer HL. Primary antiphospholipid syndrome as a new cause of autoimmune pancreatitis. Gut. 2004;**53**:468

[39] Hannu T, Mattilla L, Siitonen A, et al. Reactive arthritis attributable to Shigella infection: A clinical and epidemiological nationwide study. Annals of the Rheumatic Diseases. 2005;**64**:594-598

[40] Orlando A, Renna S, Perricone G, et al. Gastrointestinal lesions associated with spondyloarthopaties. World Journal of Gastroenterology. 2009;**15**:2443-2448

[41] Rudwaleit M, Baeten D. Ankylosing spondylitis and bowel disease. Best Practice & Research. Clinical Rheumatology. 2006;**20**:451-466

[42] Smale S, Natt RS, Orchard TR. Inflammatory bowel disease and spondylarthropathy. Arthritis and Rheumatism. 2001;**44**:2728-2736

[43] De Keyser F, Baeten D, Van den Bosch F, et al. Gut inflammation and spondyloarthropathies. Current Rheumatology Reports. 2002;**4**:525-532

[44] Yurdakul S, Tuzuner N, Yardakul I, et al. Gastrointestinal involvement in Behçet's syndrome: A controlled study. Annals of the Rheumatic Diseases. 1996;**55**:208-210

Section 5

Recent Advances in the Treatment of Faecal Incontinence

Chapter 6

Anal Injectable and Implantable Bulking Agents for Faecal Incontinence

John Camilleri-Brennan

Abstract

Faecal incontinence (FI) is a common condition, the prevalence of which increases with age. It is associated with a negative impact on the quality of one's life. The aetiology is multifactorial; hence, both the diagnosis and the treatment of faecal incontinence may be challenging. A variety of surgical treatments for faecal incontinence have emerged over the years. One of these is the use of anal bulking agents. Anal bulking agents have been available for over 25 years, with various studies being published. Initial results were disappointing, mainly due to lack of efficacy and reliability as well as concerns about safety. Great strides have been made recently with the introduction of the anal implants Gatekeeper (GK) and Sphinkeeper (SK). This chapter explores the evolution of anal injectables and implants, discusses operative techniques and provides a critical analysis of the results of the various studies to date.

Keywords: faecal incontinence, anal sphincter, anal implants, anal injectables, anal bulking agents, gatekeeper, Sphinkeeper

1. Introduction

Faecal incontinence (FI) may be defined as an impaired ability of the control of the release of flatus or faeces. It is a socially stigmatising condition that may have an adverse effect on one's quality of life. From the financial point of view, the investigation and treatment of faecal incontinence may add to a significant cost to the health systems of most countries. In fact, the annual treatment cost of patients in the UK with urinary and faecal incontinence is of about £500 million.

Many factors may be involved in the pathophysiology of FI. A thorough clinical assessment of the patient is therefore mandatory. This starts with a full history, which may include a cognitive assessment if necessary. The characteristics of the faeces and the type and frequency of incontinence should be noted. Urge incontinence is suggestive of poor external anal sphincter (EAS) function, whilst passive and post-defaecatory incontinence indicates that internal anal sphincter (IAS) function is weak. Various questionnaires that enable the clinician to quantify the degree of incontinence and the impact on quality of life are available. These include symptom-specific questionnaires, such as the ones developed by Vaizey et al. [1] and Wexner et al. [2]

and the faecal incontinence quality of life (FIQOL) scale developed by Rockwood et al. [3], and also generic questionnaires such as the Short Form 36 (SF 36) [4].

A full examination of the patient, including the abdomen and perineum and a neurological examination in some cases, is necessary. Beneficial investigations include a flexible sigmoidoscopy, anal manometry (resting and squeeze pressure), rectal compliance, pudendal nerve terminal motor latency (PNTML) and endoanal ultrasound (EAUS). Clinicians, however, need to be able to determine which test to perform, and when, as well as be able to correctly interpret the results.

The management of FI is complex and multidisciplinary, involving the general practitioner, continence nurse, physiotherapist, gastroenterologist, urologist and colorectal surgeon. Conservative measures, which include patient education and support, improvement in diet and bowel habit, judicious use of anti-diarrhoeal medication and pelvic floor exercises, are used in the first instance. This is, in fact, recommended in the UK by the National Institute for Clinical Excellence (NICE) guideline 'CG49 Faecal Incontinence' [5]. If these measures fail, surgical intervention may be necessary. A variety of surgical options are available, with the appropriate therapy being selected depending on the cause of the incontinence and the patient's cognitive function and general physical condition (**Table 1**). One of the surgical options available is the use of anal bulking agents.

1. **Restoration and improvement of residual sphincter function**
a. Correcting a defective external anal sphincter
Sphincteroplasty (end-to-end repair; overlap repair)
b. Correcting a defective pelvic floor:
Levatorplasty
Postanal repair
Total pelvic floor repair
c. Correction of anorectal deformities
d. Sacral nerve stimulation (SNS)
e. Posterior tibial nerve stimulation (PTNS)
2. **Increasing the outlet resistance of the anal sphincter**
a. Augmentation of the anal sphincter and anal cushions (anal bulking agents)
b. Anal submucosal fibrosis (SECCA)
c. Anal encirclement (Thiersch procedure)
d. Non-dynamic graciloplasty
3. **Dynamic sphincter replacement**
a. Dynamic graciloplasty
b. Artificial anal sphincter
4. **Antegrade continence enema (ACE)**
5. **Faecal diversion**
a. Colostomy
b. Ileostomy

Table 1.
Surgical options in the management of faecal incontinence.

2. Anal bulking agents

Anal bulking agents have emerged as a treatment for FI, following the success of bulking agents for urinary stress incontinence in females. In the urology setting, bulking agents have been employed to augment the bladder neck and increase urethral resistance [6]. Therefore, the aim of anal bulking agents is to prevent FI by closing the anal canal or increasing the pressure within the anal sphincter.

The ideal characteristics of a bulking agent have been described in the literature [7]. The injected or implanted substance should be biocompatible, non-migratory, non-allergenic and noncarcinogenic. The substance should also be easy to inject or implant and should produce an improvement in continence, both in the short term and in the long term.

2.1 The evidence for anal bulking agents

Anal injectables and implantables have been used to manage faecal incontinence for over 20 years. It may be useful to chart their development over the years and to classify this development into three phases. The first phase consists of the initial experimental studies that took place in the 1990s. The second phase, from about the year 2000 onwards, encompasses an increase in the number of studies using a wide variety of agents and injection techniques. The third phase features the latest generation of anal bulking agents, the implantable polyacrylonitrile, available as Gatekeeper (GK) and Sphinkeeper (SK) devices.

2.2 Initial studies: The first phase

Anal bulking agents were first described in 1993 by Shafik [8]. Shafik, an Egyptian surgeon, is considered to be a pioneer in this field. In his first study, he described the outcomes following the injection of 5 ml of PTFE (polytef/Teflon) paste in 11 patients, 7 of whom had incontinence following a lateral internal sphincterotomy for anal fissure. In another study, the same author used 60 ml of abdominal wall fat as a submucosal injection into the rectal neck at 3 and 9 o'clock in 14 patients with partial faecal incontinence [9]. Pescatori's group from Rome, Italy, reported the use of anal injection of autologous buttock fat to restore continence in one patient who had poor results following a sphincteroplasty. This patient's continence improved following repeated injections [10].

The indications for injection of the anal bulking agents in these studies were various. Most patients had passive FI, but some had urge incontinence, indicating EAS disruption. The results of these initial studies showed that continence was improved in the short term. However, the medium- and long-term results were poor, probably because of the resorption or migration of the injected material. Reinjection was necessary in order to maintain continence.

A number of safety issues were raised with these studies. Teflon could potentially cause granuloma formation and sarcomas. The injection of autologous fat as a bulking agent in urology has been implicated in fatal fat embolism and stroke.

2.3 The second phase

The second phase in the development of anal bulking agents consisted of a wide variation in the types of materials used, surgical technique and clinical indications [11]. Some of the materials used to bulk the anal sphincter were being used in urology to augment the bladder neck. Nine different types of injectable bulking agents have been used in these studies (**Table 2**).

Type of bulking agent	Commercial name(s)	Injection site	Injection route	Published studies	No. of patients
Silicone biomaterial. Polydimethylsiloxane elastomer particles suspended in a biocompatible hydrogel made of poly-N-vinyl-pyrrolidone	PTQ; Bioplastique	Intersphincteric; within IAS	Transsphincteric	21	619
Carbon-coated zirconium beads, comprised of pyrolytic carbon-coated beads suspended in a water-based carrier gel containing β-glucan	Durasphere	Submucosal	Transmucosal; transsphincteric	7	187
Spherical particles of calcium hydroxylapatite, suspended in a gel	Coaptite	Submucosal	Transsphincteric	1	10
Dextranomer microspheres and stabilised sodium hyaluronate in phosphate-buffered 0.9% sodium chloride solution	NASHA Dx, Zuidex, Solesta	Submucosal	Transmucosal	5	192
Glutaraldehyde cross-linked collagen	Contigen	Submucosal	Transmucosal	2	90
Synthetic non-particulate hydrogel consisting of water (97.5%) and cross-linked polyacrylamide (2.5%)	Bulkamid	Intersphincteric	Intersphincteric	1	5
Cross-linked porcine dermal collagen matrix	Permacol	Submucosal; intersphincteric	Transmucosal; intersphincteric	5	172
8% ethylene vinyl alcohol copolymer dissolved in dimethyl sulfoxide. A spongy solid mass forms from the solidification of the hydrophobic copolymer when the solvent diffuses away on contact with tissue fluid	Onyx34	Intersphincteric	Intersphincteric	1	21
Expandable silicone microballoons filled with a biocompatible hydrogel made of poly-N-vinyl-pyrrolidone		Submucosal	Transmucosal	1	6

Table 2.
Injectable materials used in the second phase of studies.

2.3.1 Indications

The clinical indications for which these bulking agents were used varied from study to study. These were:

- Failure of conservative management of faecal incontinence.
- Structurally intact but weak internal anal sphincter. This would be due to either primary idiopathic degeneration of the IAS or degeneration secondary to tissue disorders such as scleroderma.
- IAS damage (childbirth, haemorrhoidectomy, anal stretch, sphincterotomy) (**Figure 1**).
- Defect in the external anal sphincter.

The main indication was IAS dysfunction or disruption. Unlike the EAS, the IAS is not amenable to surgical repair.

2.3.2 Surgical procedure and technique

The bulking agents may be inserted under local, regional (anal or pudendal nerve block) or general anaesthesia. The type of anaesthesia used depends on the preference of the patient and the surgeon. The patient may be positioned in the prone (jackknife), lithotomy or left lateral positions, although the latter position may not give a satisfactory view of the anorectum to enable accurate injection. A phosphate enema is usually administered preoperatively. The procedure is usually covered by prophylactic antibiotics, such as intravenous (IV) co-amoxiclav 1.2 g, cefuroxime 750 mg and metronidazole 500 mg or gentamicin 1.5 mg/kg and metronidazole 500 mg at induction.

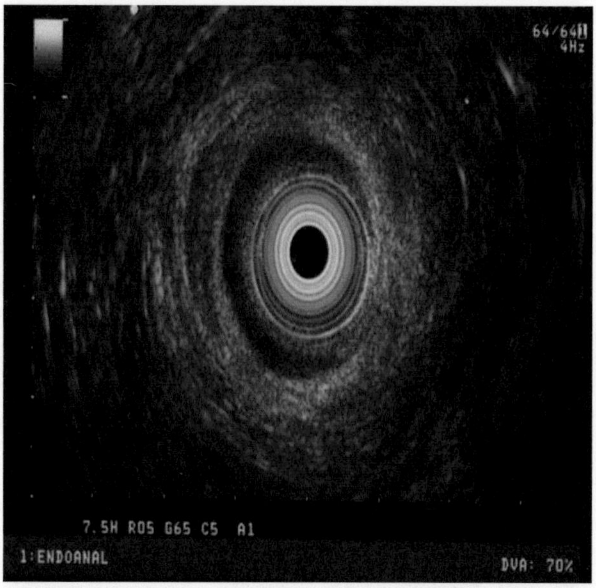

Figure 1.
Endoanal ultrasound scan showing a defect in the IAS of a 57-year-old lady with passive faecal incontinence following haemorrhoidectomy. The defect is present between the arrows from the 3 to the 5 o'clock positions.

The injection of the bulking agent varies depending on the type of substance used and the clinical indications. Three different routes of needle insertion were mentioned in the literature: transmucosal, transsphincteric or intersphincteric. The bulking agent was placed submucosally, within the intersphincteric space or within the IAS itself. For example, porcine dermal collagen (Permacol) may be injected via the transmucosal or transsphincteric route using a disposable 19G needle [12] (**Figure 2**). In patients with an intact IAS, 2.5 ml of Permacol is equally injected into the submucosal space at the 3, 7 and 11 o'clock positions above the dentate line. In cases of an IAS defect, 5 ml of Permacol may be injected at the site of the defect, with 2.5 ml of the substance injected diametrically opposite. With silicone biomaterial (PTQ or Bioplastique), four doses of 2.5 ml of silicone are used, using an 18G needle [13, 14]. Patients with an intact IAS have the silicone injected transsphincterically into the intersphincteric space at the 2, 4, 8 and 10 o'clock positions. In patients with an IAS defect, for example, after a lateral internal sphincterotomy, a total of three doses of 2.5 ml of silicone are injected into the defect. A fourth dose is injected into the intersphincteric space contralateral to the IAS defect, to provide symmetry. With carbon-coated beads (Durasphere), a total of 10 ml is injected in four divided doses in the submucosal plane using an 18G needle [14].

It is of utmost importance to ensure that the anal mucosa is not breached during injection, since that would allow intra-anal leakage of the substance. Intravascular injection must also be avoided.

Once the injection is completed, it is a good practice to leave the needle and syringe in place for a few seconds. As the needle is being withdrawn, pressure on the needle track by the index finger may prevent leakage of the bulking agent [12].

The bulking agent may be injected freehand, with an anal retractor such as Eisenhammer used to identify the IAS and intersphincteric groove. A finger placed within the anal canal may be useful to guide the needle to its correct position. However endoanal ultrasound has been recommended to guide the needle to an optimum position [13], especially if the agent is to be injected into the intersphincteric space or adjacent to a defect in the IAS.

2.3.3 Results

The majority of studies in this second phase of development were mainly case series and observational studies. Most of these studies reported either an improvement in the faecal continence scores or less frequent episodes of incontinence over time. Anorectal manometry testing is featured in some studies, with some showing an improvement in resting or squeeze pressures. Others studies showed no such improvement. Clinical improvement was not always associated with an increase in

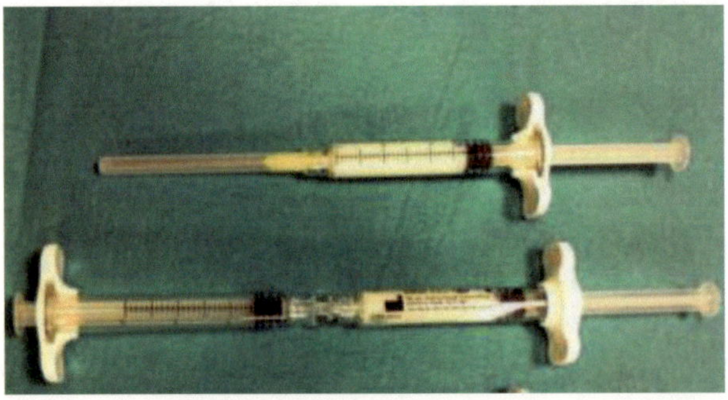

Figure 2.
Porcine dermal collagen (Permacol) in a 2.5 ml syringe.

these pressures. Quality of life was formally assessed in some of these studies. The majority reported an improvement across various domains such as physical and social function.

To date there have been 6 randomised trials using anal bulking agents, with more than 400 patients. Two trials compared a bulking agent with a sham or saline injection. Siproudhis et al. in 2007 [15] compared a silicone biomaterial (PTQ) with a normal saline injection (control) into the intersphincteric space. PTQ did not demonstrate any appreciable clinical benefit when compared to the control. The trial was however deemed to be too small to detect any differences in continence. Graf et al. in 2011 [16] compared the injection of dextranomer (NASHA Dx) against sham injection (no substance injected). Continence was better in the short term (6 months) in the active intervention group, although interestingly about 30% of patients in the control group had an improvement in their continence. This same group, the NASHA Dx study group, published the results of a prospective multicentre trial in 2014, showing that 'submucosal injection of NASHA Dx provided a significant improvement of FI symptoms in a majority of patients and this effect was stable during the course of the follow-up and maintained for 3 years'.

A small study with 10 patients by Maeda et al. in 2008 [17] revealed significant improvement at 6 weeks postinjection using injection of Bulkamid and Permacol. Continence decreased slightly in the Permacol group at 6 months. However there was no reported difference between the two agents. The numbers were too small to detect a difference. Tjandra et al. in 2009 reported the results of a randomised study comparing PTQ with carbon-coated beads (Durasphere) [14]. PTQ injection was associated with better continence scores and quality of life and was safer than Durasphere.

Tjandra et al. in 2004 reported the short-term benefits from ultrasound-guided injection of silicone biomaterial (PTQ) compared with digital guidance [13].

The follow-up for the majority of patients in studies was less than a median of 3 years. A question on the term durability and effectiveness of these agents is therefore raised. The majority (97%) of patients were only followed up once or twice. No long-term evidence on outcomes was available, and further conclusions were not warranted from the available data. None of the studies reported patient evaluation of outcomes, and thus it is difficult to gauge whether the improvement in the continence scores matched the practical symptom and quality of life improvements that mattered to the patients.

The majority of patients did not report any complications. The complications described were mainly pain, anal bruising and leakage of injected material [11, 12]. Less common complications were anal ulceration and infection (local cellulitis and abscess formation). There were two reported cases of local giant cell foreign body reaction after injection of silicone (PTQ) [18]. Durasphere has been associated with skin rashes and arthritis. Skin patch testing is therefore recommended before using this agent [14].

2.4 The third phase: The implantable gatekeeper and Sphinkeeper

A relatively new and innovative development in anal bulking technology is the Gatekeeper and Sphinkeeper (THD S.p.A., Correggio, Italy). The material used is polyacrylonitrile (Hyexpan). Polyacrylonitrile is an inert, non-allergenic, nondegradable material that is also non-immunogenic and noncarcinogenic. First developed by Medtronic in Minneapolis, USA, it was originally used as an implant in the oesophagogastric junction for the management of gastro-oesophageal reflux disease.

The main indications for the use of the GK and SK are passive faecal incontinence, secondary to IAS dysfunction or damage, where conservative measures or injection of other bulking agents such as PTQ or Permacol has failed. However, the use of GK and SK in patients with other causes of FI is being explored.

The following are contraindications to the use of the GK and SK. Similar contraindications have also been described by the product manufacturers of other anal bulking agents:

- Perianal sepsis
- Inflammatory bowel diseases with anorectal involvement (Crohn's disease, ulcerative colitis)
- Anal, rectal or colon cancer undergoing active treatment
- Rectal bleeding of unknown or undiagnosed origin
- Rectal prolapse
- Uncontrolled blood coagulation disorders
- Pelvic radiotherapy
- Immunosuppression
- Pregnancy or planned pregnancy in the next 12 months.

2.4.1 Surgical apparatus, procedure and technique

Whereas the anal bulking agents that were developed in phases 1 and 2 are injected into or around the anal canal by means of a hypodermic syringe, the Hyexpan prostheses are implanted into the intersphincteric space using a custom-made gun (**Figure 3**).

The difference between GK and SK lies in the size of the prostheses. The dehydrated GK prostheses consist of thin solid cylinders, 22 mm long and 2 mm in diameter. The success of this material depends on its hydrophilic properties.

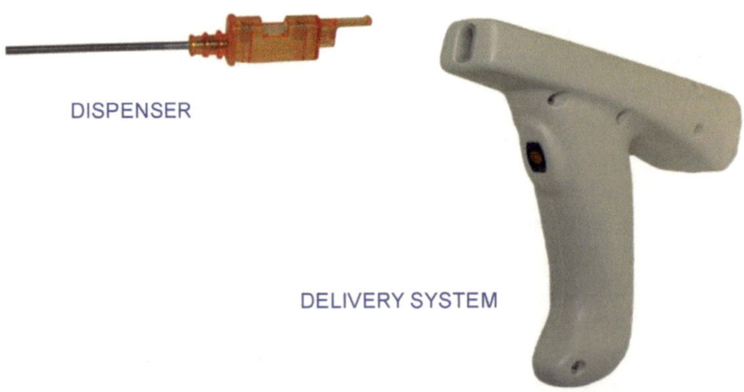

Figure 3.
The gatekeeper gun, made of the dispenser that houses one prosthesis and the delivery system. The Sphinkeeper delivery system and dispenser are similar but slightly larger.

Within 48 hours after implantation in the human tissue, the Hyexpan cylinders absorb water to become thicker and shorter. The in vitro maximum diameter is 6.5 mm and the length is 17 mm (**Figure 4**). The volume of each individual implant increases from approximately 70 mm^3 to 500 mm^3, a 750% increase. The implant also becomes much softer in consistency. On the other hand, the SK prostheses in the dehydrated state are thin, solid cylinders, 29 mm long with a diameter of 3 mm, changing their size to a length of 23 mm and a diameter of 7 mm within 48 h of contact with fluids.

The technique of implantation of the GK and SK is identical. The operation is performed under regional or general anaesthesia. Intravenous antibiotics are given at induction. The author's patients receive gentamicin 1.5 mg/kg and metronidazole 500 mg IV. The patient is placed in the lithotomy position. A strict sterile technique is used. The IAS and intersphincteric groove are identified by the placement of an anal retractor (e.g. Eisenhammer). The author's preference is a THD surgy Mini-light proctoscope, a self-illuminating anal and rectal retractor that gives a very good view of the anorectum without causing trauma to the anal sphincter (**Figure 5**). A 2 mm incision is made in the perianal skin, 2 cm from the anal verge (**Figure 6**).

Having attached the dispenser to the delivery system, the needle is inserted through the incision and tunnelled to the intersphincteric margin and introduced into the intersphincteric space. The needle is then positioned so that the tip would lie just beyond the dentate line. When the needle is identified in the correct position, by direct vision and palpation and/or by endoanal ultrasound, the prosthesis is released into the intersphincteric space (**Figure 7**).

The steps may be repeated to insert up to 10 prostheses, equidistant from each other. The GK has been originally described with the insertion of between 4 and 6 prostheses, whereas the SK has been described with the use of 10 prostheses. The choice of inserting 4 as opposed to 6 or 10 prostheses is arbitrary. The use of 10 prostheses enables the formation of a circumferential or quasi-circumferential intersphincteric ring, akin to an artificial anal sphincter. The prostheses self-fix in the desired position, thereby preventing displacement and migration in the majority of cases.

The wounds are closed with a single absorbable suture (**Figure 8**). At the end of procedure, EAUS imaging will show the location of all prostheses. The procedure takes about 30 to 40 minutes to complete and is done as a day case. Oral metronidazole 400 mg tds is prescribed for 5 days postoperatively. Oral laxatives such as lactulose are prescribed to minimise the risk of constipation. The patients are advised to avoid any anal trauma as well as anal intercourse for at least 72 h after implant insertion. The patients are followed up after 6 weeks and 3 months thereafter. The material remains identifiable both by palpation and by endoanal ultrasonography in the postoperative period (**Figures 9** and **10**).

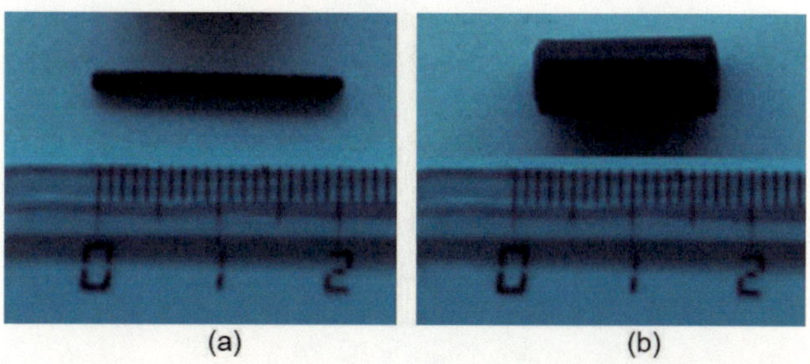

Figure 4.
(a) Shape of Hyexpan gatekeeper cylinder at insertion. (b) Fully expanded Hyexpan gatekeeper cylinder following contact with water.

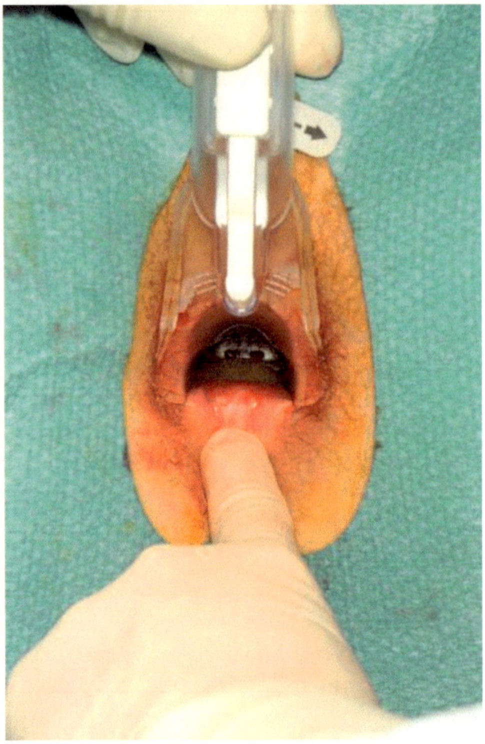

Figure 5.
Palpating the IAS and the intersphincteric groove at the 6 o'clock position with a THD surgy mini-light proctoscope in position.

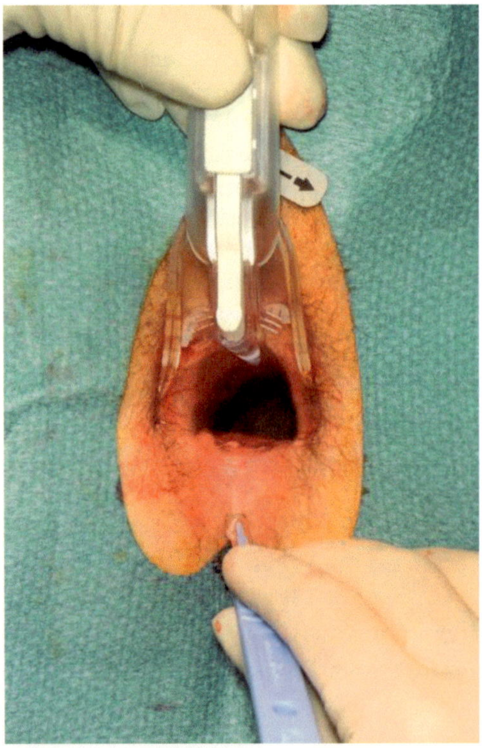

Figure 6.
Making an incision, 2 cm away from the anal verge, at the 6 o'clock position.

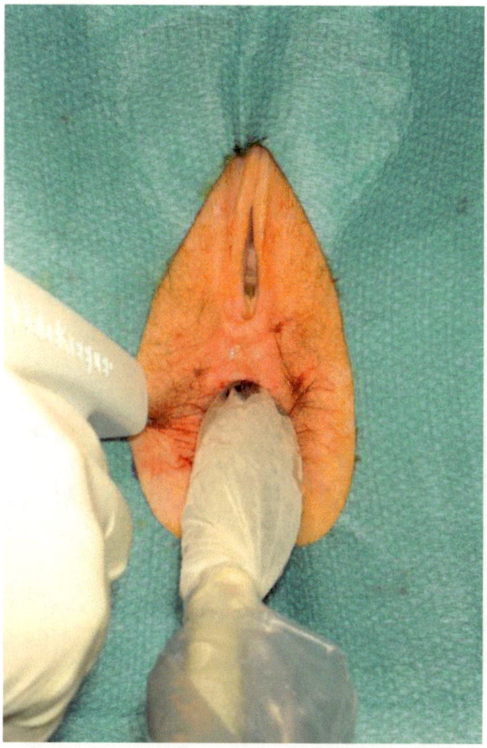

Figure 7.
The gatekeeper needle at the 9 o'clock position, with the endoanal ultrasound probe in place to determine correct placement.

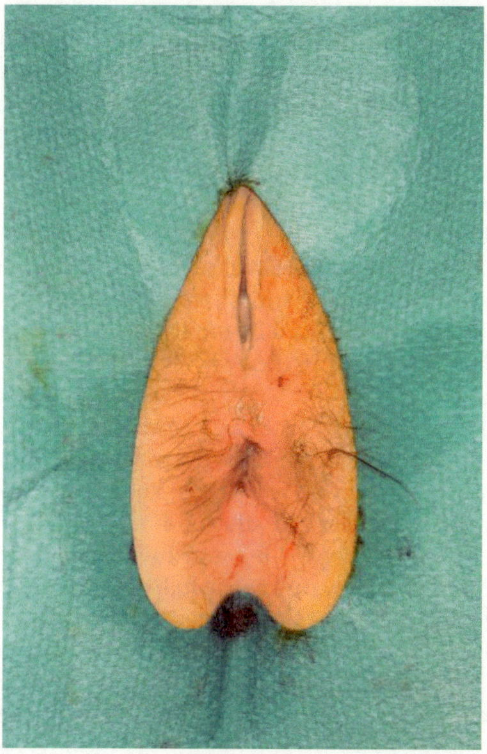

Figure 8.
Up to 10 equidistant circumferential perianal wounds, each closed with an absorbable suture (Monocryl 3/0).

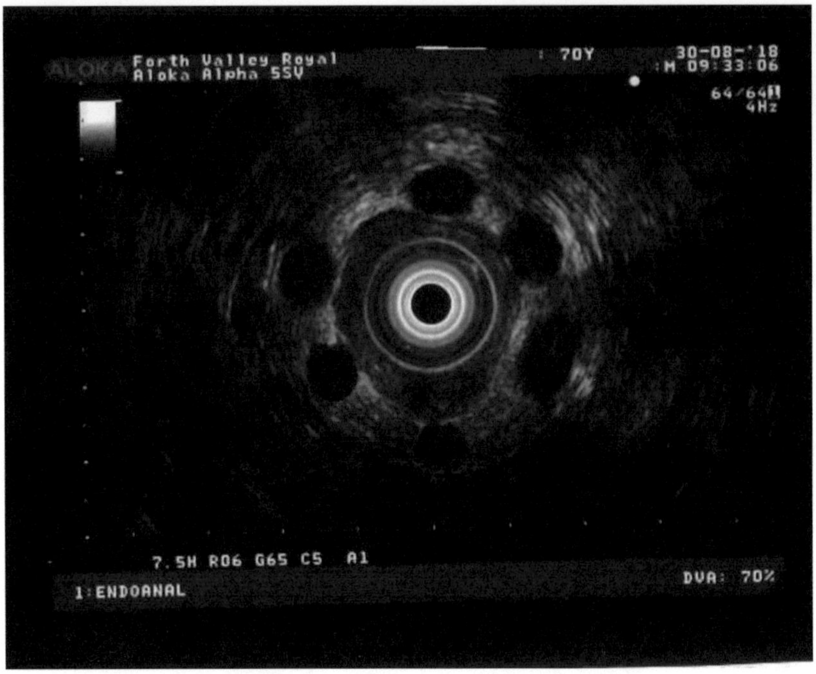

Figure 9.
Endoanal ultrasound scan (Aloka) at 6 weeks following the implantation of six gatekeeper prostheses in a 72-year-old male with idiopathic passive faecal incontinence.

2.4.2 Results

The first reported experience with the Gatekeeper was by Ratto et al. in 2011 [19]. This was a study with 14 patients. Eight had idiopathic FI, four had an IAS defect, and two had combined IAS and EAS defects. The median follow-up was of 12 months (ranging from 5 to 48 months). The authors reported a clinically significant improvement in continence in 13 patients, a sustained significant improvement in the Wexner and Vaizey scores and in the SF36 and FIQOL scores. No complications have been reported.

The second study was a comparative retrospective study by Parello et al. in 2012 [20]. Seven patients who had the Gatekeeper implanted were compared to six patients who underwent sacral nerve stimulation. The median follow-up was of 18 months in the Gatekeeper group and 20 months in the SNS group. The authors reported a sustained improvement in the Wexner continence scores with both modalities of treatment.

Fabiani et al. [21] used Gatekeeper for a group of patients affected by minor faecal incontinence. Four out of seven patients complained of passive incontinence prior to the procedure. After an average follow-up of 6 months, 6 patients reported a Wexner incontinence score under the value of 4, meaning that they rarely experienced symptoms (0 = perfect incontinence and 20 = complete incontinence). Only one patient who suffered mixed incontinence failed to respond.

Biondo et al. [22] concluded that Gatekeeper is a safe and effective procedure in more than 50% of patients for at least a year after implantation. They found that no patients had postoperative or long-term complications. Forty-eight per cent of patients were classed as responders, and significant differences were found between baseline mean Vaizey scores at 6 months, 12 months and last follow-up. At long-term follow-up (2.7 years), those patients that responded were found to have maintained an improvement more than 50% of their baseline Vaizey score.

DOI: http://dx.doi.org/10.5772/intechopen.91952

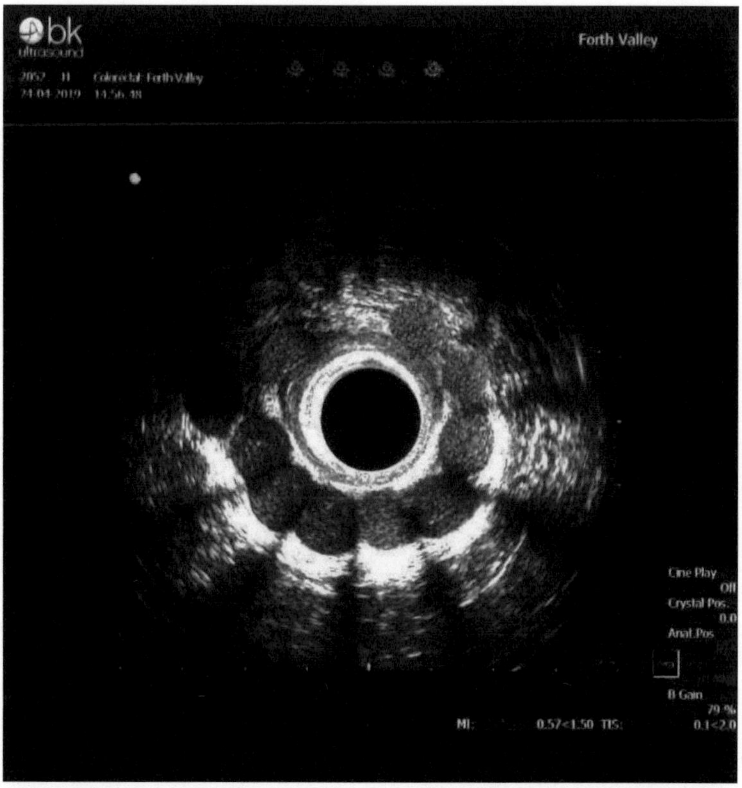

Figure 10.
Endoanal ultrasound scan (B&K) at 6 weeks following the implantation of 10 Sphinkeeper prostheses in a 68-year-old female with passive faecal incontinence and previous episiotomy.

In a multicentre study involving 54 patients and a clinical follow-up for a year, Ratto et al. [23] noted that after Gatekeeper implantation, incontinence to gas, liquid and solid stool improved significantly, soiling was reduced and the ability to defer defaecation was enhanced. All faecal incontinence severity scores were significantly reduced, and patients' quality of life improved. At 12 months, 30 patients (56 per cent) showed at least 75 per cent improvement in all faecal incontinence parameters, and 7 (13 per cent) became fully continent. Dislodgement of a few prostheses was reported, but this made no difference to postoperative continence.

The author has carried out more than 40 GK procedures in a single centre since 2012. The main indications were idiopathic FI and passive incontinence following surgery (anal stretch for anal fissure and haemorrhoidectomy). All patients had failed conservative management. There was a significant sustained improvement in the median Vaizey scores. The median (range) Vaizey scores improved from 16 (12–17) preoperatively to 5 (3–9), 4 (3–7), 4 (3–5), 4 (3–5), 5 (3–6) and 5 (3–6) at 6 weeks and at 3, 6, 12, 24 and 36 months, respectively ($p < 0.01$, Wilcoxon test). There was also an improvement in the Rockwood quality of life scores. The author reports no complications apart from minor pain that is managed by paracetamol.

Publications on the Sphinkeeper are limited. Ratto et al. [24] treated 10 patients with SK and followed them up for 3 months. The study demonstrated that the SK, with its larger prostheses than that of GK, is safe and effective. The Pelvic Floor Society of the Association of Coloproctology of Great Britain and Ireland is currently collecting prospective data on the SK from multiple centres in the UK.

3. Discussion

The development of anal injectable and implantable technology over the past 20 years has taken great strides forwards. Starting with the pioneering efforts of Shafik with autologous fat, more materials have been tried and used, the most popular being collagen (Permacol) and silicone (PTQ or Bioplastique). These agents were associated with variable and inconsistent results. Injections were frequently repeated to maintain continence in the long term. The latest generation of anal bulking agents is the implantable Hyexpan (Gatekeeper and Sphinkeeper). This material fits the criteria for the 'ideal' bulking agent. It overcomes most limitations of other bulking agents, and its use has shown very promising results.

The choice to implant the GK and SK prostheses into the intersphincteric space of the anal canal plays a key role. This location potentially avoids extrusion or migration of prostheses (different to what could happen if implanted into the submucosa). Moreover, thanks to the rapid increase of their volume, the prostheses self-fix and are unlikely to move after deployment.

The mechanism of action of anal bulking agents is a subject of debate. Most of the resting anal pressure is the function of the IAS, with some contribution from the EAS and anal cushions. Studies of faecal incontinence in patients who have undergone a traditional Milligan-Morgan haemorrhoidectomy lend support to the concept that anal cushions play an important part in the maintenance of the normal mechanism of continence. It is thought that the mechanism of action of a bulking agent injected into the submucosal space is an increase in the size of the natural anal cushions. On the other hand, a bulking agent injected or implanted into the intersphincteric space would bulk up the size of the anal sphincter. The end result would be an improvement in the seal of the lumen of the anal canal at rest and potentially an increase in resting anal pressure and in the length of the anal high pressure zone. When the injection is placed adjacent to an identifiable IAS defect, a better degree of anal canal sealing may be obtained through improvement in the configuration and symmetry of the anal canal [7]. Ratto argues that GK and SK, being embedded within the intersphincteric space, thereby pushing the EAS outwards and the IAS inwards, 'may improve sphincter contractility by increasing sarcomere length as well as increase the length of the anal canal and provide a powerful "bulking effect"' [24].

It is acknowledged that more research is required in this field. Most studies are case series with very few randomised trials. The Gatekeeper and Sphinkeeper, the latest generation of anal bulking agents, show promising results. Whether these results are maintained in the longer term or not awaits to be seen. The key factor however remains that correct patient selection is extremely important to achieve good results.

Larger series with longer follow-up and randomised controlled trials are therefore necessary. Further development on existing and emerging technology is also warranted.

Author details

John Camilleri-Brennan
Department of Surgery, Forth Valley Royal Hospital and the University of Glasgow Medical School, Scotland, UK

*Address all correspondence to: johncbrennan@doctors.org.uk

References

[1] Vaizey CJ, Carapeti E, Cahill JA, Kamm MA. Prospective comparison of faecal incontinence grading systems. Gut. 1999;**44**:77-80

[2] Jorge JMN, Wexner SD. Etiology and management of fecal incontinence. Diseases of the Colon and Rectum. 1993;**36**:77-97

[3] Rockwood TH, Church JM, Fleshman JW, et al. Fecal incontinence quality of life scale: Quality of life instrument for patients with fecal incontinence. Diseases of the Colon and Rectum. 2000;**43**(1):9-17

[4] Ware JE Jr, Sherbourne CD. The MOS 36-item short-form health survey (SF-36). I. Conceptual framework and item selection. Medical Care. 1992;**30**:473-483

[5] National Institute for Clinical Excellence (NICE). The management of faecal incontinence in adults. Clinical Guideline 49 NICE; 2007

[6] Lightner DJ. Review of the available urethral bulking agents. Current Opinion in Urology. 2002;**12**:333-338

[7] Vaizey CJ, Kamm MA. Injectable bulking agents for treating faecal incontinence. The British Journal of Surgery. 2005;**92**:521-527

[8] Shafik A. Polytetrafluoroethylene injection for the treatment of partial fecal incontinence. International Surgery. 1993;**78**:159-191

[9] Shafik A. Perianal injection of autologous fat for treatment of sphincteric incontinence. Diseases of the Colon and Rectum. 1995;**38**:583-587

[10] Bernardi C, Favetta U, Pescatori M. Autologous fat injection for treatment of fecal incontinence: Manometric and echographicassessment. Plastic and Reconstructive Surgery. 1998;**102**:1626-1628

[11] Maeda Y, Laurberg S, Norton C. Perianal injectable bulking agents as treatment for faecal incontinence in adults. Cochrane Database of Systematic Reviews. 2010;**5**:CD007959

[12] Watson NFS, Koshy A, Sagar PM. Anal bulking agents for faecal incontinence. Colorectal Disease. 2012;**14**(Suppl 3):29-33

[13] Tjandra JJ, Lim JF, Hiscock R, Rajendra P. Injectable silicone biomaterial for fecal incontinence caused by internal anal sphincter dysfunction is effective. Diseases of the Colon and Rectum. 2004;**47**:2138-2146

[14] Tjandra JJ, Chan MK, Yeh HC. Injectable silicone biomaterial (PTQ) is more effective than carbon-coated beads (Durasphere) in treating passive faecal incontinence-a randomized trial. Colorectal Disease. 2009;**11**(4):382-389

[15] Siproudhis L, Morcet J, Laine F. Elastomer implants in faecal incontinence: A blind, randomized placebo-controlled study. Alimentary Pharmacology & Therapeutics. 2007;**25**(9):1125-1132

[16] Graf W, Mellgren A, Matzel KE, Hull T, Johansson C, Bernstein M, et al. Efficacy of dextranomer in stabilised hyaluronic acid for treatment of faecal incontinence: A randomised, sham-controlled trial. Lancet. 2011;**377**(9770):997-1003

[17] Maeda Y, Vaizey CJ, Kamm MA. Pilot study of two new injectable bulking agents for the treatment of faecal incontinence. Colorectal Disease. 2008;**10**(3):268-272

[18] van Wunnik B, Driessen A, Baeten C. Local giant cell foreign body

reaction after silicone injection for fecal incontinence in humans: Two case reports. Techniques in Coloproctology. 2012;**16**:395-397

[19] Ratto C, Parello A, Donisi L, Litta F, De Simone V, Spazzafumo L, et al. Novel bulking agent for faecal incontinence. British Journal of Surgery. 2011;**98**(11):1644-1652

[20] Parello A, De Simone V, Donisi L, Litta F, Zaccone G, Ratto C. Can gatekeeper, a new bulking agent be equivalent to SNS in patients with fecal incontinence in the presence of only internal sphincter defects. Techniques in Coloproctology. 2012;**16**:77

[21] Fabiani B, Menconi CDE, Giani I, Naldini G. Anal gatekeeper a new bulking agent for faecal incontinence. Colorectal Disease;**16**(Suppl 3):37-105

[22] Biondo S, Trenti L, Noguerales F, Nomdedeu J, et al. Outcomes of gatekeeper prosthesis implantation for the treatment of fecal incontinence: A multicenter observational study. Techniques in Coloproctology. 2017;**21**:963-970

[23] Ratto C, Buntzen S, Aigner F, Altomare DF, et al. Multicentre observational study of the gatekeeper for faecal incontinence. British Journal of Surgery. 2016;**103**:290-299

[24] Ratto C, Donisi L, Litta F, Campennı P, Parello A. Implantation of SphinKeeper: A new artificial anal sphincter. Techniques in Coloproctology. 2016;**20**:59-66

Chapter 7

BioSphincter a Regenerative Medicine Approach to Treat FI

Prabhash Dadhich and Khalil N. Bitar

Abstract

A healthy sphincter physiology is a complex interplay between neural and muscle population, responsible for relaxation and contraction, which allow feces to pass and reestablishment of closure. The loss of integrity of neuromuscular functionality or cellular component results in fecal incontinence (FI). The current available treatments have been disappointing in long-term relief. This chapter represents a regenerative medicine approach to this debilitating disease, wherein a new internal anal sphincter (IAS) BioSphincter™ is bioengineered from the patient's own cells and implanted. It results in long-term restoration of the cellular integrity and reinstatement of the physiological function of the IAS. Following implantation in rodents, the engineered sphincters became vascularized and maintained their phenotype and functionality. The developed IAS BioSphincter™ were validated to treat the FI in large animals and successfully restored anorectal functionality. According to NIH/NIDDK, one out of seven people report to health care providers complaining of fecal incontinence. This chapter elucidates the long road in developing on implantable bioengineered IAS "BioSphincter™" that would benefit and improve the quality of life of a large socially distressed segment of the population.

Keywords: fecal incontinence, regenerative medicine, BioSphincters, neural progenitor cells, anorectal physiology

1. Introduction

A healthy anorectal functionality is a coordinated interplay between the enteric nervous system, smooth muscle of internal anal sphincter (IAS), striated external anal sphincter and puborectalis muscles [1]. Anomalies in any of this individual or group of tissues may lead to anorectal irregularities and diseases [2]. Fecal incontinence (FI) is devastating from a hygiene perspective due to involuntary soiling of liquid and solid stool and results in the distressing psychosocial impact on the patient [3]. Injury to the perineum may also result in the complete or partial destruction of the anal sphincter and distal rectum potentially resulting in persistent incontinence [4]. The resulting psychological stress, social stigma, decreased self-esteem and productivity can be overwhelming. In the USA, men and women suffer from FI equally with a range of 2–6% in people aged 20–30 years. The prevalence increases to over 15% in people older than 70 years [5].

Clinical characteristics of FI have been correlated with underlying sphincter pathology [1]. In the classical FI, the pelvic floor muscles are dysfunctional (due to muscle or nerve damage) and result in the frequent urge of incontinence. The urge of incontinence is mainly due to external anal sphincter defects and lower anorectal squeeze pressures. Patients with the urge of incontinence have FI episodes with awareness of the event but cannot prevent it because of the inability to increase anorectal pressures [1, 6, 7].

The passive FI caused an isolated or combined loss of smooth muscle function (IAS), skeletal muscle function (EAS), anorectal sensory mechanisms or neural control [8, 9]. It leads to loss of the sense that rectum is full and results in unknowingly leakage of stools, mucus, and flatus. Passive incontinence occurs without the patient's awareness of the event until after incontinence has occurred [6]. Patients with passive incontinence are more likely to have internal anal sphincter defects and lower anorectal resting pressures. The anal resting tone is produced by the internal anal sphincter (IAS) and the external anal sphincter. The IAS contributes 60–70% of the anal tone [10]. In addition, patients with passive incontinence have been shown to have more frequent and exaggerated IAS relaxation compared to continent controls [11]. Patients with FI have been shown to have variable loss of the Recto Anal Inhibitory Reflex (RAIR) [12].

Currently, there is no satisfactory long-term treatment for FI. Epidemiological studies indicated that most patients suffering from FI do not consult to clinicians and depend on self-management or rely on the use of adult diapers. The classical treatment of FI becomes more involved in accordance with the extent and severity of the incidences of incontinence.

Conservative management of FI is usually initiated with educating the patients with behavioral techniques. These techniques such as scheduling toileting and preventive strategies [13]. The next step is the incorporation of dietary changes using fiber supplements or laxative to normalize stool consistency [14]. Along with dietary modulations, antidiarrheal drugs, alpha (1 and 2) receptor agonists could also be used to control the frequency of FI episodes [15]. Pelvic floor muscle exercise and biofeedback are other conservative methods to manage initial stages of FI. Biofeedback methods are behavioral management that incorporates electronic and mechanical devices to emphasize bowel and muscle retraining. Pelvic floor muscle exercises with biofeedback improve sense and strength of pelvic floor muscles for contraction during rectal distention and uncontrollable urge of FI [16, 17]. According to an observational study, these conservative methods resulted in 50% reduction in the frequency of FI and 21% adequate relief in FI [13]. The effectiveness and success of these measures may help in the management of mild cases of FI.

If the patient does not improve with the mentioned conservative methods, the patient is offered advanced therapies. Advanced therapies are more invasive and involve different levels of surgical interventions such as electrical stimulation, sphincteroplasty, injection of bulking agents, and implantable devices. Sacral nerve and tibial nerve stimulation found to be more effective than electrical stimulation of muscles [18–20]. In a randomized controlled trial on patients with structurally intact and innervated sphincters, the implantation of a battery-operated stimulator was found to be effective from 36 to 50% [18, 19]. The frequency of episodes of FI was reduced during stimulation, but unaffected without stimulation or similar to sham [13]. The implantable devices such as artificial bowel sphincter [21], magnetic beads [22] and synthetic polymer rings are implanted around the anal canal to augment the pressure. There is a lack of randomized controlled trial towards long-term safety and efficacy of these procedures. The sphincteroplasties (suturing of the separated sphincter) and graciloplasty (wrapping of gracilis muscle around the anal canal) are another class of surgical procedures to treat FI. These procedures have shown varying rates of success and high chances of obstructed defecation. Inert materials (silicone elastomers, ceramic beads) or biopolymers (polycaprolactam beads) as bulking agents injected around the anal canal to increase resting pressure [23]. There was no specific success reported regarding long-term efficacy.

DOI: http://dx.doi.org/10.5772/intechopen.86345

However, a 3-month follow up study of injection of dextranomer microspheres resulted in a 50% reduction in FI frequency in 52% patients [24].

Cell delivery is advanced translation method for long-term efficacy in FI. Stem cell constructs were developed, and were able to generate smooth muscle tone but lacked innervation [25]. Autologous transplantation of muscle progenitor cells into the sphincters exhibited potentials for re-stabilization of myogenic functionality in the anal sphincters [26]. Delivery of autologous human adipose-derived stem cells in poorly functioning sphincter muscle as replacement of fibrous tissues acted as a mechanical support for physiological functions [27]. Injection of autologous myoblasts into the external anal sphincter defect also resulted as a safe and promising approach to improve symptoms of FI induced owing to obstetric anal sphincter trauma [28]. Sphincters are complex organs for cell delivery. There are several challenges to overcome in direct cell delivery, such as specific types and dosages of cells, circular distribution and orientation of cells around the anal canal after injection, functional integration with host cells and long-term effects such as biodistribution, tumorigenicity.

Current cell delivery technologies focus either on the reinstatement of the striated muscle of the external anal sphincter or mechanical support to the sphincter, with little attention on the reinstatement of IAS function [29–32]. The terminal gut function requires coordinated contraction and relaxation of the smooth muscle of rectum mediated through the enteric nervous system of IAS [2, 6]. To remedy an injured anus, it is imperative to reinstate both smooth muscle and intrinsic neural components of IAS. We describe the evolution of a regenerative medicine approach proposed to provide critical components to reinstate function in the anorectum and remedy passive fecal incontinence caused by injury to the IAS. According to this hypothesis, implantation of engineered autologous BioSphincters reinstate IAS function and restore fecal continence. Autologous smooth muscle and neural progenitor cells from gut biopsies were used to bioengineer intrinsically innervated IAS [33, 34]. Autologous functional intrinsically innervated IAS construct was successfully implanted into healthy animal models. Following implantation in rodents, the engineered sphincters became vascularized and maintained their phenotype and functionality [35–38]. A large animal model of passive fecal incontinence was developed and demonstrated sustained restoration of fecal continence, and restoration of basal tone and restoration of RAIR after implantation of engineered autologous, intrinsically innervated internal anal sphincter (IAS) BioSphincters [10, 39] (**Figure 1**).

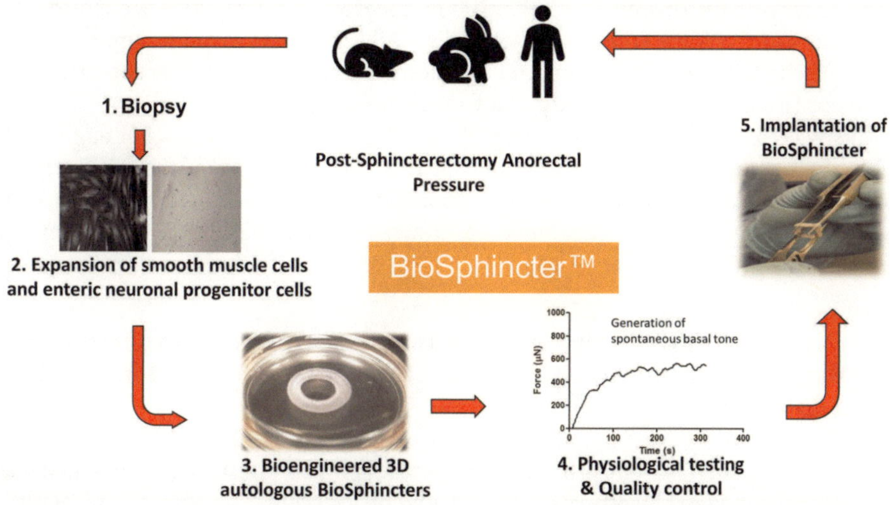

Figure 1.
Regenerative medicine approach to treat fecal incontinence using autologous bioengineered BioSphincter.

This chapter summarizes the regenerative medicine approach of bioengineering of BioSphincters, including developmental stages of the technology, challenges, process optimization, characterization, detail pre-clinical evaluation of the BioSphincter towards the treatment of FI.

This chapter encompasses both in vitro and in vivo studies designed to support the safety and efficacy of bioengineered sphincters. Studies performed in vitro include the generation of three-dimensional internal anal sphincter models using rabbit IAS smooth muscle cells and human IAS smooth muscle cells. The in vitro studies also describe the intrinsical innervation of bioengineered IAS sphincters. Studies performed in vivo are described in two parts, small animal rodent studies and a large animal, rabbit fecal incontinent model. Small animal rodent studies included: (1) generation and implantation of IAS smooth muscle cell sphincter into a C57BL/6 J rodent; (2) generation and implantation of human innervated bioengineered sphincters into an athymic rodent model, at subcutaneous and peri-anal sites. Large animal studies demonstrating successful implantation of intrinsically innervated autologous IAS BioSphincters were conducted in a rabbit model of fecal incontinent.

2. Bioengineering an in vitro three-dimensional physiological model of the internal anal sphincter from rabbit smooth muscle cells

The objective of the early studies was to develop an in-vitro three-dimensional (3-D) physiological model of the IAS smooth muscle cells. In this initial attempt, rabbit origin IAS smooth muscles were cultured on top of a loose fibrin gel; subsequently, these cells migrated and self-assembled in circumferential alignment. As the cells matured, the fibrin gel contracted around a 5-mm-diameter silicon mold, resulting in a 3-D cylindrical ring of sphincteric tissue [40].

Histological analysis exhibited a gradient of cell alignment in the bioengineered IAS sphincters. The engineered sphincters were analyzed for physiological functionality using an isometric force transducer. Constructs were placed between a stationary central pin and the measuring arm of the organ bath transducer (Harvard Apparatus, Holliston, MA). The bioengineered sphincter generated a spontaneous basal tone, and treatment with 8-bromo-cAMP (8-Br-cAMP) resulted in relaxation. In the next step, agonist-induced stimulation (using acetylcholine) resulted in calcium- and concentration-dependent peak contraction. This effect was diminished by the addition of 8-Br-cAMP. Similar bioengineered IAS sphincters were also generated using colonic smooth muscle cells. IAS constructs display significant differences in functionality compared to colonic smooth muscle cells constructs, which confirmed tissue specificity and functionally to IAS [40].

This was the first successful attempt to develop 3-D in vitro model of engineered IAS sphincters using smooth muscle cells of IAS. Bioengineered IAS sphincters displayed circular cell alignment and physiological functionality. The functionality and physiological response in engineered tissues exhibited similarity to IAS smooth muscle in vivo [38].

3. In vivo cytocompatibility and functionality analysis on subcutaneous implantation of physiologically functional bioengineered internal anal sphincter

After successful bioengineering an IAS specific sphincter tissues, the next goal was to evaluate the in vivo biocompatibility and adverse reaction. The objective of these studies was to test the post-implantation functionality of bioengineered sphincters engineered using IAS smooth muscle cells. **Table 1** summarized the detail study design.

In this endeavor, smooth muscle cells were isolated from the IAS of donor C57BL/6 mice. Smooth muscle cell constructs were engineered on Sylgard coated plates using fibrin gel, as described previously [40]. The engineered constructs were successfully implanted into the subcutaneous region of same strain mice and treated with either fibroblastic growth factor-2 or saline as controls using a micro-osmotic pump. Mice were euthanized after 4 weeks, and the implant was harvested. The implant was intact, healthy in color without any degradation, and interestingly displayed muscle attachment to the back of the mouse, with neovascularization. Constructs exhibited no external sign of inflammation, fibrosis, or infection, because of the use of syngeneic tissue. The supplement of FGF-2 also helped in tissue viability, cellular integrity, and vascularization. The harvested tissues maintained smooth muscle alignment and phenotype [37, 38].

The post-implant harvested constructs were analyzed for force generation. The harvested implants generated and maintained the spontaneous basal tone in the absence of any external stimuli. The developed tone confirmed the integrity of ionic membrane characteristics, membrane receptors and their intracellular signaling mechanisms for contraction and relaxation. On treatment of a relaxing stimulant such as a vasoactive intestinal peptide (VIP), the force and magnitude of relaxation were consistent before and after implantation. The rapid, and dose-dependent sustained (over 30 min without signs of muscle fatigue) contractions on the treatment of acetylcholine and phorbol dibutyrate was elicited as well. The physiological studies confirmed that implanted bioengineered sphincters maintain IAS physiological functionality after implantation [37, 38].

In summary, IAS sphincters using smooth muscle tissue could be bioengineered. The bioengineered sphincters were cytocompatibility, functional, without any adverse reaction and had potential to be used as a graft for dysfunctional internal anal sphincter [37, 38].

Steps	Study objective(s)	Test article	Animal model	Key outcome (e.g., safety (tumor/tox/biodistribution), efficacy, characterization, stability, degradation)
Study purpose: cell isolation				
Isolation of SMC	To isolate IAS smooth muscle cells (SMC) and characterization of smooth muscle	In vitro expanded IAS smooth muscle cells	C57BL/6J mice	Smooth muscle cells expressed cell lineage appropriate phenotype markers
Study purpose: bioengineered sphincters				
Bioengineering sphincters with smooth muscle	Characterize the bioengineered sphincters	Bioengineered sphincters	C57BL/6J mice	Formation of stable sphincters
Study purpose: implantation of bioengineered sphincters into rodent				
Implantation of bioengineered sphincters	Optimization of the implantation procedure	Bioengineered sphincters	C57BL/6J mice	Bioengineered sphincters were implanted subcutaneously on syngeneic mice (C57BL/6J) model
Study purpose: end points analysis				
Bioengineered sphincters histopathology	Analysis of fibrosis/inflammation and functional activity	Implanted bioengineered sphincters	C57BL/6J mice	No fibrosis or inflammation was observed in bioengineered sphincter implants

Table 1.
Summary of nonclinical study for safety and efficacy of bioengineered sphincters in C57BL/6J mice.

4. Bioengineering an internal anal sphincter derived from smooth muscle cells isolated from the human internal anal sphincter

The preliminary work in the previous sections using SMCs harvested from animal models confirmed the feasibility of engineering functional physiologic IAS constructs and initial biocompatibility. [40]. The next objective was to validate the feasibility of engineering IAS sphincter constructs from SMCs of human IAS origin.

Human IAS was received from NDRI and SMCs were harvested following previously described protocol. At confluency, SMCs were seeded on Sylgard coated plates with fibrin gel. Cells migrated and aligned circularly around the Sylgard mold located at the center of the plate. All the 3-D bioengineered sphincter constructs successfully formed within 5–10 days of seeding of Human IAS SMCs [34].

The developed human IAS constructs displayed the essential characteristics of a native functional IAS; the bioengineered IAS constructs able to generate the spontaneous myogenic basal tone and respond to different pharmacological agents. Bioengineered human IAS sphincters also exhibited dose-dependent force generation in response to different stimulants. The IAS smooth muscle constructs displayed a tissue-specific basal tone compared to colonic muscle cells. The basal tone, acetylcholine-induced contraction and PdBU generated were reduced by calphostin-C but not with Y-27632. The detailed functionality resulted that the protein kinase C (PKC) pathway (independent of the Rho/ROCK pathway) appeared to be responsible for IAS specific tone and contractions [34].

The process of bioengineering IAS constructs using human IAS smooth muscles was highly reproducible. The developed IAS muscle constructs were functionally similar to native IAS sphincters. This was the first report demonstrating the generation of a functional in vitro model of human IAS that may be used for the elucidation of mechanisms associated with smooth muscle sphincter myogenic malfunction and for the investigation of treatments for fecal incontinence [34].

5. Bioengineered IAS generated from human cells and preliminary biocompatibility and functional analysis after implantation in an athymic rodent model

In the previous sections, IAS muscle constructs were successfully bioengineered with animal and human origin IAS circular muscles. The bioengineered mouse IAS muscle constructs displayed physiological functionality after implantation in wild type mice. However, compare to anatomy and physiology of native IAS sphincters, the bioengineered muscle constructs lacked innervation of the neuronal population. Therefore, the next target in these studies was to intrinsically innervation of bioengineered IAS muscle constructs and evaluation of cellular viability, physiological functionality, and safety after implantation. **Table 2** summarized the detail study design.

In this effort, the human IAS muscles were harvested and cultured as described previously. The neuronal cell line was isolated from a D13 embryo from H-2Kb-tsA58 immortomouse. The bioengineering of constructs was divided into two steps. In the first step, the isolated neuronal stem cells were mixed with hydrogel and plated in the Sylgard coated plates. After gelation, IAS origin smooth muscle cells were mixed with the collagen gel and overlaid to the previous cell-hydrogel. A fully compacted sphincter-like construct were developed in the first 60 h [35].

The neuronal stem cells differentiation towards functional neurons was carried out in a specific media targeted to neural differentiation. The bioengineering

Steps	Study objective (s)	Test article	Animal model	Key outcome (e.g., safety (tumor/tox/ biodistribution), efficacy, characterization, stability, degradation)
Study purpose: cell isolation				
Isolation of SMC	To isolate IAS smooth muscle cells (SMC) and characterization	In vitro expanded IAS smooth muscle cells	Cadaver human	Smooth muscle cells expressed cell lineage appropriate phenotype markers
Isolation of neural cells from embryo of immortomouse	To isolate neural cells and characterization	In vitro expanded neural cells	h-2kb-tsA58 immortomouse	Neural cells expressed cell lineage appropriate phenotype markers
Study purpose: bioengineered sphincters				
Bioengineered Sphincters with smooth muscle and neural cells	Characterize the bioengineered sphincters	Bioengineered sphincters	Cadaver human and h-2kb-tsA58 immortomouse	• Formation of intrinsically innervated sphincters • Bioengineered sphincters exhibited basal tone, relaxation and contractile activity
Study purpose: implantation of bioengineered sphincters into rodent				
Implantation of bioengineered sphincters	Optimization of the implantation procedure	Bioengineered sphincters	RAG1−/−mice	Bioengineered sphincters were implanted subcutaneously on athymic mice (RAG1−/−) model
Study purpose: end points analysis				
Bioengineered sphincters histopathology	Analysis of fibrosis/ inflammation and functional activity	Implanted bioengineered sphincters	RAG1−/− mice	• No fibrosis or inflammation was observed in Bioengineered Sphincter implants • Harvested post-implant sphincters capable of maintaining basal tone, relaxation, and contractile activity

Table 2.
Summary of nonclinical study for safety and efficacy of bioengineered sphincters in athymic rodent model.

process took 9 days to generate an intrinsically innervated muscle constructs mimicking physiological functionality to native IAS tissues. The neural cell differentiation was further confirmed by positive expression of mature excitatory (choline acetyltransferase; ChAT) and inhibitory (VIP) motor neurons in the quantitative analysis using PCR. The cross-sections of engineered sphincters were demonstrated positive immunoreactivity against ChAT and VIP markers. After physiological functional analysis, the bioengineered sphincter were implanted subcutaneously into immune suppressed RAG1−/− mice for 4 weeks [35].

At harvest, the implanted construct exhibited neo-vascularization without any symptom of fibrosis or immunogenic reaction. The immuno-histological analysis confirmed that the sections of the harvested implant displayed reticulated neural network innervated into intact aligned muscles. The section displayed microvasculature and several blood vessels embedded within the implanted smooth muscles [35].

The myogenic and neuronal components were preserved after implantation. All the bioengineered constructs were able to generate myogenic spontaneous basal tone pre- and post-implantation. A rapid and robust relaxation response was observed against VIP. This relaxation was 50–70% attenuated on pre-treatment of TTX, indicated that VIP-induced relaxation has both neuronal, as well as myogenic component. The relaxation was further validated with EFS and resulted in transient relaxation ultimately recovered to basal tone. The inhibition of nitrergic and VIP-ergic EFS-induced relaxation (by antagonizing nitric oxide synthesis or receptor interaction) confirmed the relaxation of enteric nerves results in nitrergic as well as VIP-ergic inhibitory neurotransmission in the implants. The excitatory neurotransmitter Ach (and partial inhibition on pre-treatment with TTX)-induced contraction response emulated before and after implantation, confirmed synergistic involvement of both neuronal and myogenic components. Fundamental electromechanical coupling of smooth muscle was also maintained during implantation, rendering the implanted IAS physiologically similar to in vivo IAS [35].

This was the first attempt of bioengineering of intrinsically innervated human IAS constructs. Both of myogenic and neuronal components of constructs were stable, sustained, viable and synergistically responsive after implantation in immune-suppressed mice. The study also concluded that bioengineering of intrinsically innervated sphincter is feasible, scalable, and customizable to match specific size and cell population. This leads to one step closer towards bioengineering of human engineered BioSphincters.

6. Bioengineering of physiologically functional intrinsically innervated human internal anal sphincter constructs

In previous studies, IAS smooth muscle constructs were engineered [34, 40] and implanted for cytocompatibility and physiological analysis. These preliminary studies were proof of concept using human origin SMCs and immortomouse-origin neural stem cells. To translate the bioengineered sphincter to the clinical realm, it was essential to use human origin neural cells to engineer IAS sphincters.

The next objective was to develop bioengineering physiologically functional, intrinsically innervated human IAS tissues, using human origin neural cells and IAS muscle cells. Therefore, a method was optimized for the isolation of neuronal progenitor cells (NPCs) from intestinal biopsies of adult human donors. The cell culture and characterization protocol were standardized to yield an undifferentiated pure population of enteric neural progenitor cells [33].

Several matrix compositions were evaluated as a carrier for differentiation of adult enteric NPCs to functional neurons. The type-1 collagen with laminin was optimized as hydrogel for neural differentiation [41, 42]. The collagen acts as a matrix for mechanical strength and laminin is important for neuronal development. The SMCs has the ability to reform the collagen hydrogel into 3D structure due to matrix metalloproteinase activity [43]. During this restructure of hydrogel from 2D to 3D, SMCs came into close proximities of NPCs and enhanced the NPCs differentiation. Detail NPCs-SMCs interactions were studied, and it was observed that mature smooth muscle was essential for the direct differentiation of adult enteric NPCs [33]. The ratio of NPCs and SMCs were also studied and concluded that 200,000 NPCs/construct with 500,000 SMC/constructs were optimum do generate a native physiological response [33].

The constructs responded appropriately to physiologically relevant stimulatory and inhibitory neurotransmitters during functional analysis. It was validated in immunocytochemistry, the intrinsically innervated bioengineered construct exhibited excitatory and inhibitory motor neuronal population. The constructs displayed characteristics of functional mature contractile IAS smooth muscle as well. Overall, the human innervated functional IAS sphincter like tissues were successfully bioengineered and characterized [33].

7. Peri-anal implantation of bioengineered human internal anal sphincter constructs intrinsically innervated with human neural progenitor cells

After successful bioengineering of human IAS sphincter-like tissues, it was essential to evaluate the in vivo safety and functionality. In the next part of the study, a method was developed for isolation of rectal verge in an athymic rodent

Steps	Study objective (s)	Test article	Animal model	Key outcome (e.g., safety (tumor/tox/biodistribution), efficacy, characterization, stability, degradation)
Study purpose: cell isolation				
Isolation of SMC	To isolate IAS smooth muscle cells (SMC) and characterization	In vitro expanded IAS smooth muscle cells	Cadaver human	Smooth muscle cells expressed cell lineage appropriate phenotype markers
Isolation of neural progenitor cells	To isolate neural progenitor cells and characterization	In vitro expanded neural progenitor cells	Cadaver human	Neural progenitor cells expressed cell lineage appropriate phenotype markers
Study purpose: bioengineered sphincters				
Bioengineered sphincters with smooth muscle and neural progenitor cells	Characterize the bioengineered sphincters	Bioengineered sphincters	Cadaver human	• Formation of intrinsically innervated sphincters • Bioengineered sphincters exhibited basal tone, relaxation, and contractile activity
Study purpose: implantation of bioengineered sphincters into rodent				
Implantation of bioengineered sphincters	Optimization of the implantation procedure	Bioengineered sphincters	athymic nude rats	Bioengineered sphincters were implanted peri-anal site on athymic nude rats model
Study purpose: end points analysis				
Bioengineered sphincters histopathology	Analysis of fibrosis/inflammation and functional activity	Implanted bioengineered sphincters	athymic nude rats	• No fibrosis or inflammation was observed in Bioengineered Sphincter implants • Harvested post-implant sphincters capable of maintaining basal tone, relaxation, and contractile activity

Table 3.
Summary of nonclinical study of safety and efficacy of peri-anal implantation of human origin bioengineered sphincters into athymic rodent model.

model. Athymic nude mice were larger animal compared to normal mice. The selection of immune deficient rat for implantation studies of human-origin bioengineered constructs was to avoid any immune rejection.

The intrinsically innervated human IAS Sphincter were bioengineered using IAS origin SMCs and enteric NPCs. The developed surgical models were used to implant bioengineered sphincter into the perianal region of athymic rats for 4 weeks, following assessment of viability and functionality [36]. All the rats survived till respective time points without any obstruction or difficulty with defecation or fecal accumulation. Histopathology analysis concluded the absence of any abscess formations, infection, or adverse reaction. The implanted constructs were stable and intact at perirectal tissue of the rat, without any sign of fibrosis or neoplasia. Immuno-histological analysis with endothelial-specific antigen, von Willebrand's factor confirmed neovascularization and formation of several blood vessels. The contractile smooth muscle phenotype was maintained by exhibiting positive expression to human reactive muscle specific antibodies. **Table 3** summarized the detail study design [36].

Pre- and post-implant physiological force measurement studies confirmed distinct characteristics like native sphincters. The engineered IAS sphincter exhibited stable spontaneous myogenic basal tone. There was a robust response to different relaxant and excitatory stimulants, which was persistent after implantation.

This study concluded that for clinical application the bioengineered sphincter could be used in an additive manner rather than in a replacement manner, where native compromised IAS sphincter can be supported by transplantation of additional bioengineered sphincters. In this way, the patient's own IAS can be preserved and augmented with additional autologous functional neuro-muscular components [36].

8. Long-term non-clinical study of autologous bioengineered BioSphincters for the treatment of fecal incontinence

This study aimed to provide data for a large animal model in support of the use of Bioengineered sphincter as a new therapy to treat FI. These nonclinical studies were conducted to test the safety and efficacy of using autologous cell bioengineered sphincters as a regenerative medicine approach for treating induced FI in rabbits. The study design consisted of four steps. **Table 4** summarizes the four steps including their objectives and key outcomes.

8.1 Selection of a large animal model for nonclinical studies of fecal incontinence

Currently, there is no model for FI where the defect is specific to the internal anal sphincter. In humans, the IAS is responsible for 70% of anal basal pressure, anal closure, and fecal continence. The New Zealand white rabbit (female, 3.0–3.5 kg at the enrollment of the study) was chosen as an animal model because the anatomy and the surgical planes of the anal area are similar to humans. The rabbit was selected as a good model for successful identification and surgical resection of full thickness biopsies with a successful outcome. Thus, the rabbit is a good large animal model for our lab to utilize in evaluating FI. The number of animals, experimental protocols, and overall study design used in this study were reviewed and approved by the Wake Forest Institutional Animal Care and Use Committee before conducting any component of this study involving animals. Each rabbit was given a unique identification number that was printed on the cage card. Each rabbit was identified using a unique identification number. All data collected on each animal was referenced with the unique animal identification number and tattooed onto the

Steps	Study objective(s)	Test article	Animal model	Key outcome (e.g., safety (tumor/tox/biodistribution), efficacy, characterization, stability, degradation)
Study purpose: developing FI model and autologous cell isolation				
IAS hemi-sphincterectomy	To induce FI	Donor IAS tissue	Female New Zealand rabbits	Lack of fecal hygiene and significant reduction in anal basal pressure and RAIR
Isolation of SMC	To isolate autologous IAS smooth muscle cells (SMC) characterization of autologous smooth muscle	In vitro expanded IAS smooth muscle cells	Female New Zealand rabbits	Smooth muscle cells expressed cell lineage appropriate phenotype markers
Small intestinal biopsy	To isolate neural progenitor cells (NPC) characterization of autologous NPC	In vitro expanded small intestine neural progenitor cells	female New Zealand rabbits	Neural progenitor cells expressed cell lineage appropriate phenotype markers
Study purpose: autologous bioengineered sphincters				
Bioengineered sphincters with autologous smooth muscle and neural progenitor cells	Characterize the bioengineered sphincters	Autologous bioengineered sphincters	female New Zealand rabbits	Restoration of fecal hygiene, anal basal pressure, and RAIR
Study purpose: implantation of engineered autologous bioengineered sphincters to treat FI in rabbits				
Implantation of bioengineered sphincters	Optimization of the implantation procedure	Autologous bioengineered sphincters	female New Zealand rabbits	The dosage of bioengineered sphincters was optimized four bioengineered sphincters were implanted on each rabbit in the treated group
Anal basal pressure and RAIR	Effects of bioengineered sphincters on the restoration of continence	Autologous bioengineered sphincters	female New Zealand rabbits	Rabbits with induced FI receiving bioengineered sphincter implants had anal basal pressure, and RAIR restored to normal baseline, but rabbits with induced FI in the non-treated group and sham surgery group had consistently reduced anal basal pressure and RAIR
Study purpose: end points analysis				
Blood results	Effects of implants on blood cell counts, kidney and liver function, and electrolytes.	Implanted bioengineered sphincters	female New Zealand rabbits	There were no adverse effects of implants on blood values
Tissue pathology	Effects of experimental conditions on tissue pathology	Implanted bioengineered sphincters	female New Zealand rabbits	There were no effects of experimental condition on local or peripheral histopathology

Steps	Study objective(s)	Test article	Animal model	Key outcome (e.g., safety (tumor/tox/ biodistribution), efficacy, characterization, stability, degradation)
Clinical presentation	Morbidity/mortality	Implanted bioengineered sphincters	female New Zealand rabbits	There were no effects of bioengineered sphincter implantation on morbidity or mortality
IAS histopathology	Fibrosis/inflammation	Implanted bioengineered sphincters bioengineered sphincter	female New Zealand rabbits	No definitive difference between bioengineered sphincter implants and naïve. No evidence of neoplasia

Table 4.
Summary of nonclinical study of safety and efficacy of bioengineered sphincters.

ear of each animal to prevent mix-up. Rabbits were acclimated for at least 6 days before enrollment in the study [10, 39].

8.2 Study groups

The groups of the study, summarized in **Table 5**, was developed to assess the post-implantation safety of bioengineered sphincters in rabbits at three-time points (3, 6, and 12 months). All animals underwent IAS hemi-sphincterectomy to induce FI. Rabbits were randomly divided into three experimental groups: (1) non-treated group (incontinent control), (2) treated group (received surgical implantation of bioengineered sphincters 6–8 weeks following sphincterectomy through a surgical opening of the anal verge), and (3) Sham surgery group (surgical opening of the anal verge was performed followed by immediate closure without implantation of bioengineered sphincters).

8.2.1 Development of FI

The IAS hemi-sphincterectomy was performed on all the rabbits to induce passive FI. The development of passive FI was confirmed in each assessment of fecal hygiene and anorectal pressure. Baseline manometry readings were obtained on all rabbits before any surgeries. Following hemi-sphincterectomy, anorectal manometry was performed on all rabbits to confirm passive FI, which was identified by lack of fecal hygiene and by a significant decrease in anal basal pressure and RAIR in all rabbits [10, 39].

8.2.2 Bioengineering of autologous BioSphincters

The SMCs were isolated from the IAS harvested during hemi-sphincterectomy. Isolated cells were characterized by α-smooth muscle actin and smoothelin markers. Cells stained positive confirming contractile phenotype of smooth muscle cells. NPCs were isolated from small intestine biopsies. Cells were then characterized by immunofluorescence and stained positive for p75NTR, Nestin, and Sox2, confirming neural crest-derived stem cells. Both cell types were expanded for 4 weeks to obtain the required number to form the bioengineered sphincters.

Intrinsically innervated IAS sphincters were bioengineered using both types of cells as described previously. Bioengineered sphincter products were characterized using different methods. The presence of aligned smooth muscle cells and the

DOI: http://dx.doi.org/10.5772/intechopen.86345

Study groups (no. of rabbits)	Baseline manometry	Sphincterectomy to induce FI	Manometry post sphincterectomy	4–6 weeks post sphincterectomy	1 month	3 months	6 months	12 months
Non-treated group (11)	✓	✓	✓	No treatment	Manometry post sphincterectomy			
Treated group (10)	✓	✓	✓	Implant bioengineered sphincters	Manometry post implant			
Sham surgery group (5)	✓	✓	✓	Sham surgery	Manometry post sham			

Table 5.
Study groups for the non-clinical study.

differentiated functional neural network was confirmed via immune-reactivity against smoothelin and βIII tubulin. These results further validated via positive expression of smoothelin and βIII tubulin qPCR. Engineered IAS sphincters were tested for physiological functionality. The engineered tissues able to generate the spontaneous basal tone and exhibited a robust stable response following pharmacological or electrical stimuli. The bioengineered autologous BioSphincters were implanted adjacent to IAS tissues into the respective rabbits [10, 39].

8.2.3 Implantation and restoration of fecal continence

Anorectal manometry is a technique used to measure contractility in the anus and rectum. Anorectal manometry was performed initially at baseline prior to any surgery. These measurements reflected the control state for all animals in this study. Anorectal manometry was performed prior to any surgery (before animals went for any procedure) to record the baseline, and 1 month following IAS hemi-sphincterectomy (biopsy), then at 3, 6, and 12 months in each experimental group.

8.2.3.1 Restoration of anorectal pressure

IAS hemi-sphincterectomy resulted in a significant decrease in anal basal pressure and RAIR compared to baseline (no surgery), supporting the validity of the induced-incontinence model. In the sham surgery group, anal basal pressure and RAIR were not improved and were comparable to readings from rabbits in the non-treated group. Compared to baseline, the basal pressure in non-treated and sham group was decreased by 41% ($p < 0.0001$) after 1 month of hemi-sphincterectomy and remained low up to study time point of 12 months. Similarly, RAIR was also reduced by 50.9% from the baseline ($p < 0.0001$). It remained low in non-treated group (49.2%) and sham groups (40.0%) compared to baseline till the study time point.

This reduced anorectal functionality was restored within 1-month post-implantation of autologous BioSphincters in the treated group. The resting pressure was returned to baseline after 4 weeks of implantation and remained similar up to 12 months. RAIR was restored by ~88% in initial 1 month and improved within 3 months and sustained till 12 months. The restoration of basal pressure and RAIR were significantly higher ($p < 0.0001$) than values observed in the non-treated group and sham groups.

8.2.3.2 Improvement in fecal hygiene

The IAS hemi-sphincterectomy affected fecal hygiene of the rabbits. This was evident from messy rabbit cages as feces were dispersed over the whole area of the cage. There was a definite lack of anal area hygiene as the area was always covered in a thin layer of feces. After implantation, the fecal hygiene returned to normal with a clean anal area and normal defecatory movement.

An improvement in defecatory activity was observed as early as 3 weeks after implantation of the bioengineered sphincters. Stool consistency returned to a firm pellet, similar to what was observed before FI was induced by the sphincterectomy.

8.2.3.3 Histopathology assessment

The post-implant harvested tissues displayed intact BioSphincter after 12 months of implantation. The presence of a thick continuous sheet of muscles innervated with neuronal network validated the manometry outcomes. There was the absence of any

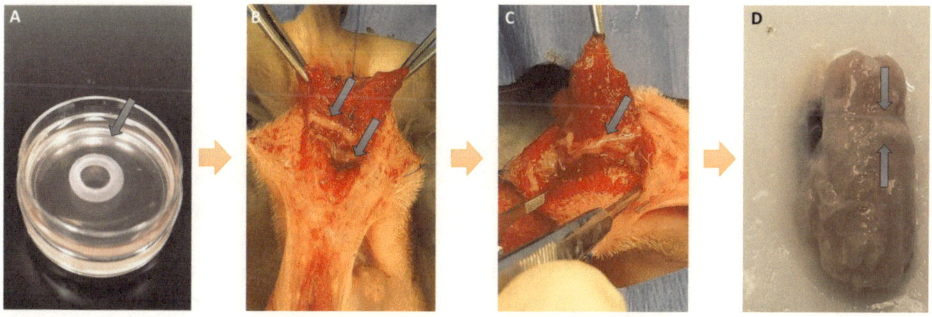

Figure 2.
Different stages from bioengineered sphincter to implantation; (A) bioengineered sphincter; (B) implantation of two bioengineered sphincters; (C) 4 implanted bioengineered sphincters; and (D) implanted bioengineered sphincter after euthanasia (after 12 months of implantation).

fibrosis or avascular collagen around the implant, indicating no foreign-body reaction with the implants. Pathologic findings in this study were generally minor and consisted primarily of a low incidence of background changes and minor changes attributable to implantation. There was no evidence of neoplasia. These results confirmed that the bioengineered sphincters were viable and functional in vivo with the maintenance of both the muscle and neural components [10, 39].

In this study, passive Fi was successfully developed in the large animal model. The bioengineered intrinsically innervated IAS constructs from the autologous cells retrieved at biopsy. The IAS constructs were bioengineered and implanted after 6–8 weeks after harvesting the cells (**Figure 2A**); then, one by one, four bioengineered sphincters were implanted at the anal site (**Figure 2B**). The four bioengineered sphincters were stacked together at the site (**Figure 2C**). After 12 months of implantation, implanted bioengineered sphincters appeared intact as one tissue at the site (**Figure 2D**).

The animals resumed normal activity and defecatory bowel movement. There was no indication of any rectal outlet obstruction or anal stenosis. Anorectal manometry was performed on the animals monthly beginning 6 weeks after implantation. The animals exhibited a reinstated basal tone and RAIR. Animals were maintained and monitored up to 12 months after implantation. At each endpoint, after euthanasia, the harvested implant was tested. Results show that the construct maintained physiological functionality. The tests show that both muscle and neural type of cells maintained their physiological function. In other experiments, we have demonstrated that the cells of the implant stayed within the implant and did not migrate outside the location of the implant.

9. Conclusion

Regeneration of an intrinsically innervated function IAS sphincter is a promising approach for long-term relief from passive FI. The IAS muscle and neural cells synergized in collagen-laminin hydrogel as a 3D sphincter like architecture, mimicking the native IAS cell orientation and innervation. The bioengineering process has been optimized, scaled up for clinical application using human origin cells. The signaling pathways for sphincter tone and contraction were characterized. The bioengineered sphincter able to generate spontaneous tone and response to different pharmacological agents was comparable to human IAS. The stability, viability and cytocompatibility analysis of engineered sphincters were carried out in vitro and in vivo conditions. The step-wise pre-clinical assessment of engineered autologous BioSphincters confirmed biocompatibility as IAS sphincter substitute, without any adverse effect. The implanted autologous BioSphincters vascularized, integrated with the impaired native IAS and regenerated stable, circularly oriented IAS muscle population, innervated with the neural network. The regeneration approach provided immediate symptomatic relief by restoration fecal hygiene. We have developed a large animal model of passive fecal incontinence and demonstrated sustained restoration of fecal continence, and restoration of basal tone and restoration of RAIR in this model after implantation of engineered autologous intrinsically innervated internal anal sphincter (IAS) BioSphincters. In a clinical scenario, this innovative approach will be able to reinstate continence, by providing an additive functional intrinsically innervated IAS bioengineered from the patient's cells.

As summary, regeneration, and implantation of the IAS BioSphincter will benefit a large socially distressed segment of the population via restoration of physiological function of the IAS, resolve FI, and improving quality of life.

Acknowledgements

This work was supported by NIH/NIDDK STTR R42DK105593.

Conflict of interest

KNB is the founder of CELLF BIO LLC a startup biotech that has an interest in developing treatments for neurodegenerative diseases of the gut.

Author details

Prabhash Dadhich[1,2] and Khalil N. Bitar[1,2,3,4]*

1 Wake Forest School of Medicine, Wake Forest Institute for Regenerative Medicine, Winston Salem, NC, USA

2 Program in Neuro-Gastroenterology and Motility, Wake Forest School of Medicine, Winston Salem, NC, USA

3 Section on Gastroenterology, Wake Forest School of Medicine, Winston Salem, NC, USA

4 Virginia Tech-Wake Forest School of Biomedical Engineering and Sciences, Wake Forest School of Medicine, Winston Salem, NC, USA

*Address all correspondence to: kbitar@wakehealth.edu

References

[1] Rao SS. Pathophysiology of adult fecal incontinence. Gastroenterology. 2004;**126**(1 Suppl 1):S14-S22. DOI: 10.1053/j.gastro.2003.10.013

[2] SSCC R, Bharucha AE, Chiarioni G, et al. Anorectal disorders. Gastroenterology. 2018;**150**(6): 1430-1442.e4. DOI: 10.1053/j.gastro.2016.02.009

[3] Bartlett L, Nowak M, Ho Y-H. Impact of fecal incontinence on quality of life. World Journal of Gastroenterology. 2009;**15**(26): 3276-3282

[4] Lazarescu A, Turnbull GK, Vanner S. Investigating and treating fecal incontinence: When and how. Canadian Journal of Gastroenterology. 2009; **23**(4):301-308. Available from: http://www.ncbi.nlm.nih.gov/pmc/articles/PMC2711681/

[5] Goode PS, Burgio KL, Halli AD, et al. Prevalence and correlates of fecal incontinence in community-dwelling older adults. Journal of the American Geriatrics Society. 2005;**53**(4): 629-635. DOI: 10.1111/j.1532-5415.2005.53211.x

[6] Engel AF, Kamm MA, Bartram CI, Nicholls RJ. Relationship of symptoms in faecal incontinence to specific sphincter abnormalities. International Journal of Colorectal Disease. 1995; **10**(3):152-155. DOI: 10.1007/BF00298538

[7] Bharucha AE. Pelvic floor: Anatomy and function. Neurogastroenterology and Motility. 2006;**18**(7):507-519. DOI: 10.1111/j.1365-2982.2006.00803.x

[8] Rattan S. The internal anal sphincter: Regulation of smooth muscle tone and relaxation. Neurogastroenterology and Motility. 2005;**17**(Suppl 1):50-59. DOI: 10.1111/j.1365-2982.2005.00659.x

[9] Bharucha AEA, Dunivan G, Goode PPS, et al. Epidemiology, pathophysiology, and classification of fecal incontinence: State of the science summary for the National Institute of Diabetes and Digestive and Kidney Diseases (NIDDK) workshop. The American Journal of Gastroenterology. 2015;**110**(1):127-136. DOI: 10.1038/ajg.2014.396

[10] Bohl JL, Zakhem E, Bitar KN, Autonomic I, Neurological N. Successful treatment of passive Fecal incontinence in an animal model using engineered Biosphincters: A 3 month follow-up study. Stem Cells Translational Medicine. 2017;**6**(9):1795-1802. DOI: 10.1002/sctm.16-0458

[11] Huebner M, Margulies RU, Fenner DE, et al. Age effects on internal anal sphincter thickness and diameter in nulliparous females. Diseases of the Colon and Rectum. 2007;**50**(9):1405-1411. DOI: 10.1007/s10350-006-0877-7

[12] Lindsey I, Jones OM, Smilgin-Humphreys MM, Cunningham C, Mortensen NJ. Patterns of fecal incontinence after anal surgery. Diseases of the Colon and Rectum. 2004;**47**(10):1643-1649

[13] Whitehead WE, Rao SSC, Lowry A, et al. Treatment of fecal incontinence: State of the science summary for the National Institute of Diabetes and Digestive and Kidney Diseases workshop. The American Journal of Gastroenterology. 2015;**110**(1):138-146. DOI: 10.1038/ajg.2014.303

[14] Bliss DZ, Jung HJ, Savik K, et al. Supplementation with dietary fiber improves fecal incontinence. Nursing Research. 2001;**50**(4):203-213. DOI: 10.1097/00006199-200107000-00004

[15] Omar MI, Alexander CE. Drug treatment for faecal incontinence in

adults. Cochrane Database of Systematic Reviews. 2013;(6):1-61. DOI: 10.1002/14651858.CD002116.pub2

[16] Heymen S, Scarlett Y, Jones K, Ringel Y, Drossman D, Whitehead WE. Randomized controlled trial shows biofeedback to be superior to pelvic floor exercises for fecal incontinence. Diseases of the Colon and Rectum. 2009;**52**(10):1730-1737. DOI: 10.1007/DCR.0b013e3181b55455

[17] Norton C, Chelvanayagam S, Wilson-Barnett J, et al. Randomized controlled trial of biofeedback for fecal incontinence. Gastroenterology. 2003; **125**(5):1320-1329. DOI: 10.1053/S0016-5085(03)01368-4

[18] Leroi AM, Siproudhis L, Etienney I, et al. Transcutaneous electrical tibial nerve stimulation in the treatment of fecal incontinence: A randomized trial (CONSORT 1a). The American Journal of Gastroenterology. 2012; **107**(12):1888-1896. DOI: 10.1038/ajg.2012.330

[19] Tan E, Ngo N-T, Darzi A, Shenouda M, Tekkis PP. Meta-analysis: Sacral nerve stimulation versus conservative therapy in the treatment of faecal incontinence. International Journal of Colorectal Disease. 2011;**26**(3):275-294. DOI: 10.1007/s00384-010-1119-y

[20] Hull T, Giese C, Wexner SD, et al. Long-term durability of sacral nerve stimulation therapy for chronic fecal incontinence. Diseases of the Colon and Rectum. 2013;**56**(2):234-245. DOI: 10.1097/DCR.0b013e318276b24c

[21] Wong MTC, Meurette G, Wyart V, Glemain P, Lehur P-A. The artificial bowel sphincter: A single institution experience over a decade. Annals of Surgery. 2011;**254**(6):951-956. DOI: 10.1097/SLA.0b013e31823ac2bc

[22] Lehur P-A, McNevin S, Buntzen S, Mellgren AF, Laurberg S, Madoff RD. Magnetic anal sphincter augmentation for the treatment of fecal incontinence: A preliminary report from a feasibility study. Diseases of the Colon and Rectum. 2010;**53**(12):1604-1610. DOI: 10.1007/DCR.0b013e3181f5d5f7

[23] Luo C, Samaranayake CB, Plank LD, Bissett IP. Systematic review on the efficacy and safety of injectable bulking agents for passive faecal incontinence. Colorectal Disease. 2010;**12**(4):296-303. DOI: 10.1111/j.1463-1318.2009.01828.x

[24] Mellgren A, Matzel KE, Pollack J, Hull T, Bernstein M, Graf W. Long-term efficacy of NASHA Dx injection therapy for treatment of fecal incontinence. Neurogastroenterology and Motility. 2014;**26**(8):1087-1094. DOI: 10.1111/nmo.12360

[25] Singh J, Rattan S. Bioengineered human IAS reconstructs with functional and molecular properties similar to intact IAS. American Journal of Physiology. Gastrointestinal and Liver Physiology. 2012;**303**(6):G713-G722. DOI: 10.1152/ajpgi.00112.2012

[26] Kajbafzadeh A-M, Elmi A, Talab SS, Esfahani SA, Tourchi A. Functional external anal sphincter reconstruction for treatment of anal incontinence using muscle progenitor cell auto grafting. Diseases of the Colon and Rectum. 2010; **53**(10):1415-1421. DOI: 10.1007/DCR.0b013e3181e53088

[27] Sarveazad A, Newstead GL, Mirzaei R, et al. A new method for treating fecal incontinence by implanting stem cells derived from human adipose tissue: Preliminary findings of a randomized double-blind clinical trial. Stem Cell Research & Therapy. 2017;**8**(1):40. DOI: 10.1186/s13287-017-0489-2

[28] Frudinger A, Kolle D, Schwaiger W, Pfeifer J, Paede J, Halligan S. Muscle-derived cell injection to treat anal incontinence due to obstetric trauma: Pilot study with 1 follow-up.

Gut. 2010;**59**(1):55-61. DOI: 10.1136/gut.2009.181347

[29] Tan JJY, Chan M, Tjandra JJ. Evolving therapy for fecal incontinence. Diseases of the Colon and Rectum. 2007; **50**(11):1950-1967. DOI: 10.1007/s10350-007-9009-2

[30] Pathi SD, Acevedo JF, Keller PW, et al. Recovery of the injured external anal sphincter after injection of local or intravenous mesenchymal stem cells. Obstetrics and Gynecology. 2012;**119**(1): 134-144. DOI: 10.1097/AOG.0b013e3182397009

[31] Jorge MJN, Wexner SD. Etiology and management of fecal incontinence. Diseases of the Colon and Rectum. 1993;**36**(1):77-97. DOI: 10.1007/BF02050307

[32] White AB, Keller PW, Acevedo JF, Word RA, Wai CY. Effect of myogenic stem cells on contractile properties of the repaired and unrepaired transected external anal sphincter in an animal model. Obstetrics and Gynecology. 2010;**115**(4):815-823. DOI: 10.1097/AOG.0b013e3181d56cc5

[33] Gilmont RR, Raghavan S, Somara S, Bitar KN. Bioengineering of physiologically functional intrinsically innervated human internal anal sphincter constructs. Tissue Engineering. Part A. 2014;**20**(11–12): 1603-1611. DOI: 10.1089/ten.tea.2013.0422

[34] Somara S, Gilmont RR, Dennis RG, Bitar KN. Bioengineered internal anal sphincter derived from isolated human internal anal sphincter smooth muscle cells. Gastroenterology. 2009;**137**(1): 53-61. DOI: 10.1053/j.gastro.2009.03.036

[35] Raghavan S, Gilmont RR, Miyasaka EA, et al. Successful implantation of bioengineered, intrinsically innervated, human internal anal sphincter. Gastroenterology. 2011;**141**(1):310-319. DOI: 10.1053/j.gastro.2011.03.056

[36] Raghavan S, Miyasaka EA, Gilmont RR, Somara S, Teitelbaum DH, Bitar KN. Perianal implantation of bioengineered human internal anal sphincter constructs intrinsically innervated with human neural progenitor cells. Surgery. 2014;**155**(4): 668-674. DOI: 10.1016/j.surg.2013.12.023

[37] Hashish M, Raghavan S, Somara S, et al. Surgical implantation of a bioengineered internal anal sphincter. Journal of Pediatric Surgery. 2010; **45**(1):52-58. DOI: 10.1016/j.jpedsurg.2009.10.010

[38] Raghavan S, Miyasaka EA, Hashish M, et al. Successful implantation of physiologically functional bioengineered mouse internal anal sphincter. American Journal of Physiology. Gastrointestinal and Liver Physiology. 2010;**299**(2):G430-G439. DOI: 10.1152/ajpgi.00269.2009

[39] Zakhem E, Bohl JL, Tamburrini R, et al. Therapeutic potential of lab-grown autologous BioSphincters for the treatment of fecal incontinence in a long-term pre-clinical study. Advanced Research in Gastroenterology & Hepatology. 2019;**12**(4):555845

[40] Hecker L, Baar K, Dennis RGRRG, Bitar KN. Development of a three-dimensional physiological model of the internal anal sphincter bioengineered in vitro from isolated smooth muscle cells. American Journal of Physiology. Gastrointestinal and Liver Physiology. 2005;**0656**(2):188-196. DOI: 10.1152/ajpgi.00335.2004

[41] Rego SL, Raghavan S, Zakhem E, Bitar KN. Enteric neural differentiation in innervated, physiologically functional, smooth muscle constructs is modulated by bone morphogenic protein 2 secreted by sphincteric smooth